Designing for Inclusion

Patrick Langdon · Jonathan Lazar ·
Ann Heylighen · Hua Dong
Editors

Designing for Inclusion

Inclusive Design: Looking Towards the Future

Springer

Editors
Patrick Langdon
Department of Engineering
University of Cambridge
Cambridge, UK

Jonathan Lazar
College of Information Studies
University of Maryland
College Park, MD, USA

Ann Heylighen
Department of Architecture
KU Leuven
Leuven, Belgium

Hua Dong
School of Design and Creative Arts
Loughborough University
Loughborough, UK

ISBN 978-3-030-43864-7 ISBN 978-3-030-43865-4 (eBook)
https://doi.org/10.1007/978-3-030-43865-4

This Springer imprint is published by the registered company Springer Nature Switzerland AG
The registered company address is: Gewerbestrasse 11, 6330 Cham, Switzerland

Preface

The Cambridge Workshop on Universal Access and Assistive Technology (CWUAAT) is a series of workshops, which is held every two years at Fitzwilliam College in Cambridge University. This volume, *Designing for Inclusion: Inclusive Design; Looking towards the Future,* comes from the 10th workshop in this series which was planned to take place in Cambridge in March 2020 but was cancelled due to COVID-19.

The CWUAAT series of workshops have celebrated a long history of cross-disciplinarity, including design disciplines, computer scientists, engineers, architects, ergonomists, ethnographers, ethicists, policymakers, practitioners and user communities. This reflects the wider increasing realisation over the long duration of the series that design for inclusion is not limited to technology, engineering disciplines and computer science but instead requires a cross-disciplinary approach. The key to this is providing a platform upon which the different disciplines can engage and see each other's antecedents, methods and points of view. The main sections of this book reflect themes that we have identified on that basis in the emerging field of design for inclusion:

I Reconciling Usability, Accessibility and Inclusive Design:
The most difficult challenge for the field—CWUAAT has contributed in this area by fostering papers that encompass multiple disciplines and perspectives;

II Designing Inclusive Assistive and Rehabilitation Systems:
A traditional area for CWUAAT—there is still, and always will be, a necessity to tackle inclusion-related problems such as capability restriction and recovering of function after injury; CWUAAT is proud to present studies on sleepwear and co-creation;

III Measuring Product Demand and Peoples' Capabilities:
A key requirement for inclusive design is good data on capabilities whether functional, social or psychological;

IV Designing Cognitive Interaction with Emerging Technologies:
Still a challenging area for inclusion, thinking encompasses self-reflection as well as interaction design;

V Designing Inclusive Architecture: Buildings and Spaces:
Now an established area for CWUAAT, this continues to reflect society whether from a child's perspective, or in transportation;

VI Data and Inclusion, User Profiling:
Quantification is vital for future inclusive design, and new metrics are continually evolving;

VII Accessibility Barriers:
There are hidden impacts to inclusion, such as time wasted on poor Web design and biases evident in interviewing techniques that deprecate the disabled.

CWUAAT has always aimed to be inclusive in the fields that it invites to the workshop. We must include social science, psychologies, anthropologies, economists, politics, governance and business. This requirement is now energised by imminent new challenges arising from techno-social change. In particular, artificial intelligence, wireless technologies and the Internet of things generate a pressing need for more socially integrated projects with operational consequences on individuals in the built environment and at all levels of design and society. Business cases and urgent environmental issues such as sustainability and transportation should now be a focus point for inclusion in an increasingly pressing global context.

This book contains the reviewed papers from CWUAAT 2020 that were invited for oral presentation. The papers that have been included were selected by peer review carried out by an international panel of currently active researchers. The chapters forming the book represent a unique sample of current national and international researches in the fields of inclusive and architectural design, universal access, engineering design, HMI, and assistive and rehabilitative technology.

CWUAAT no longer simply represents the older notions of universal access and assistive technology although those lie at the core of the workshop. Arguably, looking back across the ten book series, it has achieved its goal of integrating a far wider community and beginning the process of integrating usability, accessibility and inclusive design. We must look forward to the future to see where this transdisciplinarity may take us.

We would like to thank all those authors and researchers who have contributed to CWUAAT 2020 and to the preparation of this book. We would also like to thank the external reviewers who took part in the review process. Many thanks are due to the reviewing members of the Programme Committee who have renewed their intention to support the workshop series. We are grateful to the staff at Fitzwilliam College for their patience and help. We must also thank the contribution of images for the cover as follows:

All cover photographs—Megan Strickfaden, University of Alberta, Canada.

March 2020

Patrick Langdon
Jonathan Lazar
Ann Heylighen
Hua Dong

Contents

List of Contributors

M. Annemans Department of Architecture, Research[X]Design, KU Leuven, Leuven, Belgium

C. Barber School of Art, Design and Architecture, University of Huddersfield, Huddersfield, UK

L. Begley School of Design and Creative Arts, Loughborough University, Loughborough, UK

M. Bradley Cambridge Engineering Design Centre, University of Cambridge, Cambridge, UK

A. Burns Catapult Solutions Ltd., Gillingham, Dorset, UK

J. Chakraborty Towson University, Towson, MD, USA

P. J. Clarkson Cambridge Engineering Design Centre, University of Cambridge, Cambridge, UK

V. d'Auria Department of Architecture, OSA, KU Leuven, Leuven, Belgium

R. Davies Catapult Solutions Ltd., Gillingham, Dorset, UK

H. Dong School of Design and Creative Arts, Loughborough University, Loughborough, UK

D. Van Dyck Faculty of Medicine and Health Sciences, Department of Movement and Sport Sciences, Ghent University, Ghent, Belgium

J. Eales Department of Human Ecology, University of Alberta, Edmonton, AB, Canada

J. Fast Department of Human Ecology, University of Alberta, Edmonton, AB, Canada

C. Fiorentino Department of Human Ecology, University of Alberta, Edmonton, AB, Canada

G. A. Giannoumis Department of Computer Science, Oslo Metropolitan University, Oslo, Norway

J. Goodman-Deane Cambridge Engineering Design Centre, University of Cambridge, Cambridge, UK

M. Griffith Trace Center, HCIL, College of Information Studies, University of Maryland, College Park, MD, USA

J. Harding WSP, Member of Wolfson College, Cambridge, RIBA, Cambridge, UK

A. Heylighen Department of Architecture, Research[x]Design, KU Leuven, Leuven, Belgium

A. Jembu Rajkumar Trace Center, HCIL, College of Information Studies, University of Maryland, College Park, USA

Y. Jiang College of Design and Innovation, Tongji University, Shanghai, China

J. B. Jordan Trace Center, HCIL, College of Information Studies, University of Maryland, College Park, USA

P. M. Langdon Cambridge Engineering Design Centre, University of Cambridge, Cambridge, UK

J. Lazar Trace Center, HCIL, College of Information Studies, University of Maryland, College Park, MD, USA

G. Lee University of Leeds, Leeds, UK

T. C. Lee College of Design and Innovation, Tongji University, Shanghai, China

L. Liu College of Engineering, Nanjing Agricultural University, Nanjing, China; School of Design and Creative Arts, Loughborough University, Loughborough, UK

L. Liu College of Design and Innovation, Tongji University, Shanghai, China

Q. Y. Liu College of Design and Innovation, Tongji University, Shanghai, China

M. Martin Department of Human Ecology, University of Alberta, Edmonton, AB, Canada

P. Nguyen Department of Architecture, Research[x]Design, KU Leuven, Leuven, Belgium; Faculty of Architecture and Planning, National University of Civil Engineering, Hanoi, Vietnam

J. Nyhof-Young Department of Family and Community Medicine, University of Toronto, Toronto, ON, Canada

E. Owusu Towson University, Towson, MD, USA

C. Paupini Department of Computer Science, Oslo Metropolitan University, Oslo, Norway

C. Ramioul Osar Architecten, Antwerp, Belgium

P. A. Rodgers Imagination, Lancaster University, Lancaster, UK

K. Schaefer School of Fashion, Ryerson University, Toronto, ON, Canada

M. Smyth School of Art, Design and Architecture, University of Huddersfield, Huddersfield, UK

M. Strickfaden Department of Human Ecology, University of Alberta, Edmonton, AB, Canada

T. Tang University of Leeds, Leeds, UK

S. Tullio-Pow School of Fashion, Ryerson University, Toronto, ON, Canada

P. Tutenel Department of Architecture, Research[x]Design, KU Leuven, Leuven, Belgium

S. Waller Cambridge Engineering Design Centre, University of Cambridge, Cambridge, UK

B. Wentz Shippensburg University, Shippensburg, PA, USA

S. Westland University of Leeds, Leeds, UK

E. Winton Imagination, Lancaster University, Lancaster, UK

E. Zitkus School of Art, Design and Architecture, University of Huddersfield, Huddersfield, UK

Reconciling Usability, Accessibility and Inclusive Design

Towards Design and Making Hubs for People Living with Dementia

E. Winton(✉) and P. A. Rodgers

Imagination, Lancaster University, Lancaster, UK
{e.winton,p.rodgers}@lancaster.ac.uk

Abstract. This paper reports on the authors' Arts and Humanities Research Council (AHRC) funded work that is developing and implementing innovative design interventions that encourage people living with dementia to remain creatively active, promote dignity, and encourage independence. This work examines how the integrative, inclusive, and collaborative actions of co-design and design disruption as theoretical approaches, involves people living with dementia in rethinking and reshaping or circumventing existing forms of dementia care. Moreover, this work seeks to change mind-sets and extant prejudiced ideas about what people living with dementia might be capable of undertaking. The inclusive activity of collaboratively designing with people who are not designers themselves, seeks to challenge and alter preconceived ideas about the capabilities of people living with dementia. The paper highlights a number of innovative interventions showing how people living with dementia can be empowered by design and how they can be supported in informing conditions where their personal identity, values, knowledge, skills, experiences, perspectives and thoughts are integral to the production of new ideas and ways of thinking and doing co-design.

1 Introduction

The UK has an ageing population where there are now more people aged over 65 than those under the age of 16. The impact of this creates increased pressures on the National Health Service (NHS), and on local and regional health and social care services. Key concerns in regards to this aging population include the prevalence of the five most common chronic conditions among the over 65s – arthritis, heart disease, stroke, diabetes and dementia – with the latter expected to increase 25% by 2020 and more than 50% by 2050. In order to counteract the increasing pressures of aging health and mental healthcare issues current government policy aims to encourage people to remain active, engage in regular exercise and refrain from behaviours that could have a detrimental effect on their health. This research focuses on developing and implementing innovative design interventions, that seek to encourage people to remain active, promote dignity, and encourage independence particularly for people living with dementia.

2 The Wicked Problem of Dementia

Supporting people as they age, in particular people living with dementia, involves the design and production of various tools, devices, systems and services that are multi-faceted, holistic and interdisciplinary in nature. These activities comprise diverse parties

P. Langdon et al. (Eds.): CWUAAT 2020, *Designing for Inclusion*, pp. 3–12, 2020.
https://doi.org/10.1007/978-3-030-43865-4_1

and stakeholders, overlapping disciplines and specialists. The degenerative nature of dementia requires that these solutions and interventions must be adaptable to progressive changes. In regards to dementia what makes the situation all the more difficult is that no two individual's journeys are the same and therefore there can be no singular prescribed approach. Instead, the nature of support requires insights where parties from various backgrounds converse and, most importantly, act to help to alleviate tensions, strains or blocks and create a valued quality of life (Phillips 2006). Family members, clinicians, support workers, and the person living with dementia need to work together to develop tailored responses to each person's situation that can ensure personhood (Kitwood 1997). As Cross (2011) articulates, design is a human activity derived to respond to human behaviours and requirements and for making novel and informed solutions. As such, designers are well placed for working in challenging areas such as supporting people living with dementia. It is here that the designer's ingenuity for making things such as service, product and spatial designs, and intervening to improve the status quo is increasingly being incorporated into health and social care contexts (Muratovski 2016).

The work in this paper looks at how the inclusive and collaborative approaches of co-design (Scrivener 2005) and design disruption (Rodgers and Tennant 2014) involve and empower people living with dementia to rethink and reshape or circumvent conventional approaches to their personal dementia care. Moreover, this work seeks to change mind-sets and existing prejudiced ideas about what people living with dementia might be capable of doing. The activity of collaboratively designing with people who are not designers themselves seeks to challenge and alter preconceived ideas about the capabilities of people living with dementia. In this work, co-design is used as a facilitating proposition that supports people to act and respond independently and collectively. Here, people living with dementia inform activities of designing through personal engagement, knowledge, insight and emotional sensibilities that may have been disregarded as a result of their diagnosis. They are then invited to act upon these insights and responses through further design actions. This work shows how people are empowered by design, how they find ways to inform a situation or be supported in informing conditions where their personal identity, values, knowledge, skills, experiences, perspectives and thoughts are integral to the production of new designed ways of thinking and doing. The thinking being particularly important in forming propositions, responding to opportunities and decision making that leads to new realities through self-efficacy (Cervone 2000).

3 Towards Design and Making Hubs for People Living with Dementia

Designed with Dementia encompasses a suite of design projects that have been undertaken with people who are living with dementia in collaboration with Alzheimer Scotland. The projects cover a number of inclusive creative processes and explorations into how we can use design thinking and making to unlock and reveal personal and collective capabilities, utilising and stimulating interests and arranging new ways of doing things. Essential to this approach is the idea that design is a social activity and as such forms a space for shared enjoyment and fun in safe experimental conditions (Rodgers and Tennant 2014). Here, each person's input is valued and any failure is not seen as problematic or undermining but as a positive part of the process or something to be learned from and responded to. The authors have undertaken a variety of projects to develop, reveal and present designed solutions with and by people living with dementia. These projects have helped "shake things up" through their actions that highlight their capabilities, individually and collectively and that direct projects with people who do not have a diagnosis of dementia. The resultant thought-provoking outcomes challenge assumptions, which have also developed people living with dementia's self-esteem and confidence through personal experiences.

Throughout these projects, design kits, tools and devices have been developed to further ongoing conversations and to build the importance of those individuals taking part. Within this work the most important actions have come from open and fun conversations that lead to creative and productive actions. The importance of this work lies in how people living with dementia have been able to form ideas, develop solutions and propose new designs for public appreciation, consumption or use. The Designed with Dementia projects highlighted in this chapter include 75BC and a Glasgow Stained-Glass Window. Both of which have used collaborative design processes to create new artefacts, where individual and collective actions have demonstrated participants' self-efficacy. The projects range from intimate small group-focussed practices through to larger projects that have engaged in excess of 200 people who are living with dementia across the UK. The public impact of there designs has resulted in excess of 1000 people visiting and buying the designed artefacts in new pop up Designed with Dementia shops.

4 Designed with Dementia: 75BC

The Designed with Dementia intervention, 75BC, is a collaborative design project that explores representations of the Glaswegian comedian Billy Connolly (Winton and Rodgers 2019). Inspired by visits to the 75BC Exhibition at the People's Palace, Glasgow and to the American artist Tschabalala Self's exhibition at the Tramway Gallery, Glasgow the group developed an idea of what Connolly meant to them and how those thoughts might be represented, which resulted in the design of new fabrics and products. What occurred in delivery of their ideas was a co-design approach that became recognisable as a typical design process. At the core of this process were discussions, decisions and creative actions undertaken with all of the participants in an open forum that included a series of stages:

- **Stage 1** Primary research where the participants used digital cameras to photograph artworks focussing on composition, structure and other attributes.
- **Stage 2** Use of a kit that repurposed Tschabalala Self's processes, participants created new representations of Connolly based on their data collection and views.
- **Stage 3** Create new pattern representations of Billy Connolly from the unexpected arrangements in Stage 2.
- **Stage 4** New 75BC patterns were printed in various scales on paper where four were selected and produced as prototypes in heavyweight cotton.
- **Stage 5** The group chose to create a range of interior products (e.g., lights, cushions, rug, bed linen, a sofa and lounge chair) in the new textiles (Fig. 1).

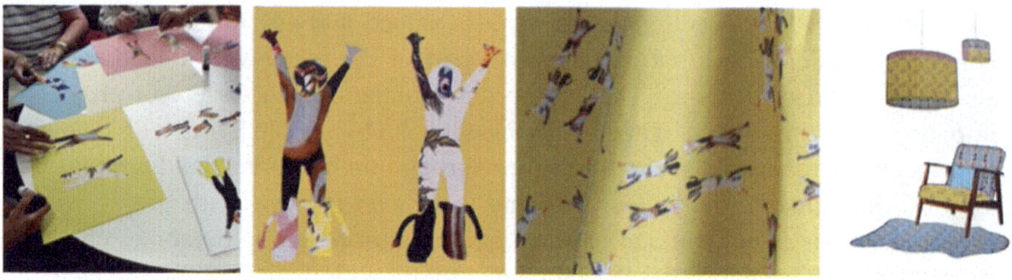

Fig. 1. The processes and results of designing and applying the 75BC fabrics

The 75BC designs, along with other participatory resources the group had co-designed featured in a public engagement event in Lancaster in March 2018. Here, over 200 people explored the group's designs and engaged in creative textile design activities. The impact included changing perspectives of those who visited, generating new understanding of the capabilities of people living with dementia.

5 Designed with Dementia: Glasgow Stained-Glass Window

This Designed with Dementia project included excursions to the Scotland Street Museum, Glasgow designed by Charles Rennie Mackintosh and to St Mungo's Museum of Religious Life and Art, Glasgow. During both visits, the importance to Glasgow of Mackintosh and his influence on contemporary stained-glass design formed a significant part of the group's discussions. This encouraged them to explore further the design of stained-glass artefacts through a collaborative workshops that included:

- **Stage 1** Photographs were taken of Mackintosh's designs and the group took part in a stained-glass workshop using different techniques such as using pre-cut tiles of colour and stained-glass colouring pens.
- **Stage 2** Production of a prototype Mackintosh-style pendant light using lighting gels and stained-glass panels, and pens to explore pattern designs.
- **Stage 3** The theme of this session was the Glasgow coat of arms. The participants collaged elements of transparent line drawings and texts in order to generate their own layouts.
- **Stage 4** Development of the ideas that emerged in earlier workshops using black printed transparencies that the group could arrange to form a collective image, which became the basis of their new stained-glass design.
- **Stage 5** The final image was scanned and produced as a transparent design for the participants to colour using acrylic paint (Fig. 2).
- **Stage 6.** Reflection has led the group to define new possibilities for their stained-glass design, which has resulted in preliminary designs for a new light.

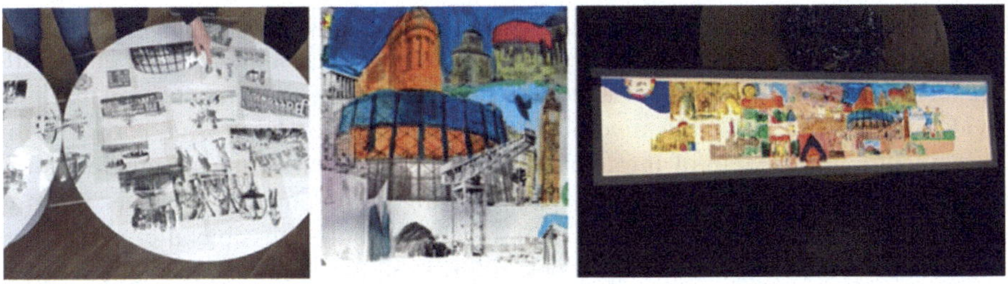

Fig. 2. Prototyping the stained glass window for Glasgow

Framed within a backlit panel the work is now presented as existing somewhere between an artwork of the city and a prototype design of a stained glass window. Using similar design processes, people living with dementia have designed and generated ceramic products including a set of hand decorated plates based on Sophie Cave's 'Floating Heads' at the Kelvingrove Museum, Glasgow and a set of travel postcards based upon the Riverside Museum, Glasgow.

6 Designed with Dementia: Pop Up Shops

As this work moves towards the creation of inclusive design and making hubs for people living with dementia, the authors have pilot-tested the idea in a number of Designed with Dementia pop up shops in Glasgow, Lancaster and Edinburgh. Each pop up shop is unique showcasing an array of designs created by people living with dementia. Each Designed with Dementia pop-up shop runs for several days, located in an existing (unused) retail space in the city centre, showcasing and selling a wide variety of uniquely designed items created through workshops such as those described in the previous sections of this paper. The Designed with Dementia pop up shops clearly illustrate how design plays a key role in empowering people living with dementia by helping to improve their decision making, greater social interaction, and personal achievements whilst supporting those individuals to work as part of a larger creative collective.

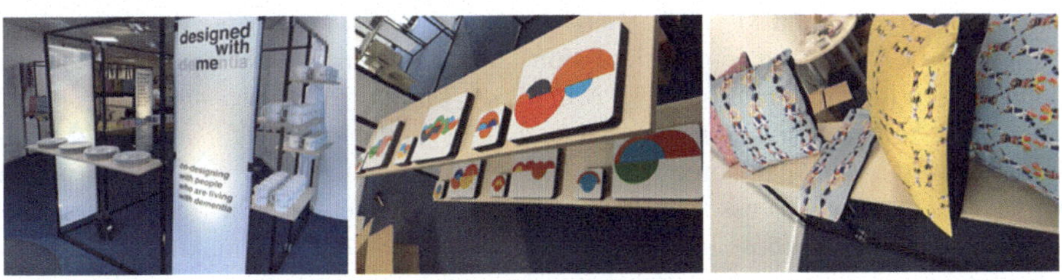

Fig. 3. Designed with Dementia pop up shops

The pop up shops have showcased and sold products such as table-ware, tote bags, mugs, coasters, aprons, ties and pencil cases (Fig. 3). All of these designed products have been designed by people living with dementia. This has involved creating artwork, making design decisions on scale, repeat patterns, material choices, and creative direction. These activities involve knowledge and skills that professional graphic and textile designers draw on in their day-to-day work. The Designed with Dementia pop up shops provide an inclusive and innovative platform to witness first-hand what people living with dementia are capable of through the design work created, manufactured, exhibited, and disseminated. We show how people living with dementia can offer much to society and we hope to change public thinking about what is possible after a diagnosis of dementia. In some of the pop up shops, it has been possible for the public to make artefacts using toolkits that have been developed by people living with dementia.

7 Analysis

A range of positive comments have been made by the co-designers (people living with dementia), their carers, and their family members throughout every stage of the design projects described in this paper. These comments have driven key activities in the projects that have been undertaken. A selection of some of the co-designers' comments made during these projects is shown in Fig. 4.

These comments clearly articulate positive feelings on the design activities conducted and they suggest value in the design exploration work. Equally important here is the voice that each participant (co-designer) has had in making decisions that have informed the design outcomes and key influences within each project. The suite of Designed with Dementia projects described here were conceived to support and nurture the opinions and decision making of the co-designers (people living with dementia). A significant consideration within all of the projects has been that the design sessions must be enjoyable and must offer a safe space for diverse ideas to formulate where differing opinions can occur. The responses and feedback collected from the co-designers during the series of co-design projects described in this paper are rich and informative. In a reflection session after the pop up shop in Glasgow, one group stated: *"I thought that was absolutely brilliant"* (Participant 1) *"It was, it really was… I thoroughly enjoyed making whatever, but I still didn't think it was good enough to sell kinda thing."* (Participant 2) *"And it was"* (Participant 1) *"It definitely was"* (Participant 3) *"It certainly made you feel quite good."* (Participant 2) *"It's good for your morale and good for your confidence."* (Participant 3) *"Thats the thing about it, is what you value you canna buy."* (Participant 1). During the co-design sessions, the co-designers were happy and felt confident to assert their opinions openly: "*Nah it's no' for me…*", "*It gave me the creeps…*", "*No. I know how it's been done, and it's been done well, but I don't like it*", "*but that's the one I want*" were just some of the phrases collected as the co-designers (people living with dementia) discussed various project tasks and actions. The rich discussion of what the shop meant to those involved along with the clear decision making and creative understanding collected in the workshops shows value in nurturing personal assertion of people living with dementia through design activities. In the co-design process and review of a wide variety of outcomes verbal, written and artefact feedback has been collected that talks of empowerment and challenges recognised aspersions which are best described by one group in the statement *"A lot of people come in think we just sit here we don't do anything. People with dementia can do great things."*

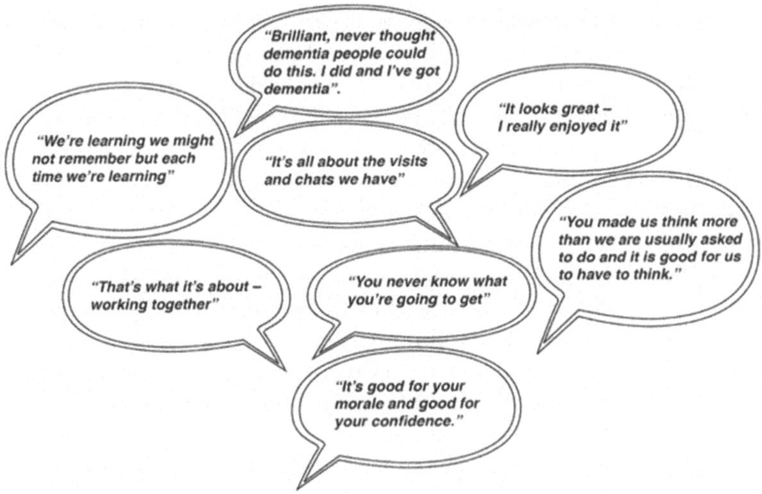

Fig. 4. A selection of co-designers' comments made during the projects

Furthermore, during the workshops, pop-up shops, public engagement events, and exhibitions of the co-designed work the value of what has been designed and exhibited has been ascertained through a number of means including feedback commentary cards and "share your thoughts" prompts. This has allowed the authors to collect diverse sets of opinions, perceptions, and comments from the general public about what might be important in terms of how we view people living with dementia and their place in wider society (Fig. 5).

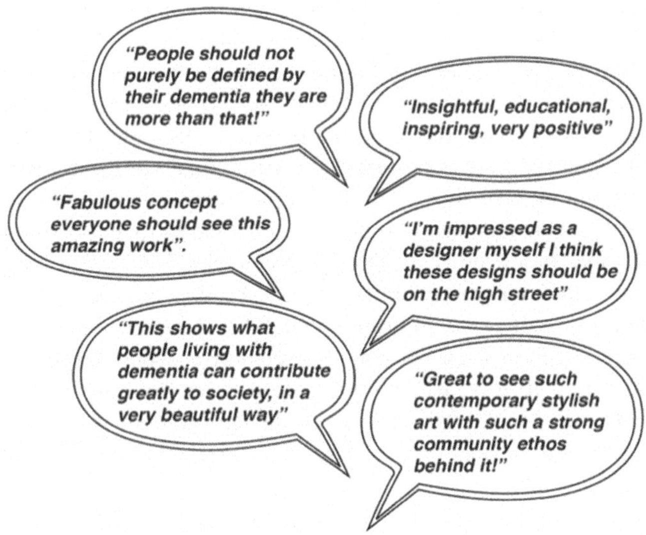

Fig. 5. Comments made by members of the public during the design projects

A large number of the feedback commentaries talked of personal experiences of dementia and the unexpected nature of what had been seen, interacted with and even bought within the pop ups. Included in these views was the recognition that at the centre of the activity was individual and collective capabilities: *"A very inspiring project, It puts the person first rather than their dementia"*. The feedback, in the main, focusses upon what is seen as uplifting responses to the stories and products: *"It's really great that this is the outcome and that it is all really different"*.

The impact of what these interventions have done is difficult to measure and comprehend but significantly the fact that the public have bought products, embedded with stories, that will exist within their homes and will form points of discussion. Where the income generated by these products will further support the designers who created them in future care and activities. During this work it is evident that our "open-doors" policy in these design and making hubs for people living with dementia reduce the closed off experience of normal dementia support centres. The welcoming environments aim to engage all aspects of society but happen to put people living with dementia at the forefront of the environment through presence or imbedded practices and objects. In doing so the approach of creating discussion, sales and action spaces might support the high street to fill voids with community focussed charitable offerings. By filling empty spaces within shopping centres – the centres benefit from rates alleviation and the centres can create more community focussed and dementia aware environments.

8 Why Are These Interventions Important?

All of the co-design projects presented in this paper have afforded a large number of people living with dementia opportunities to use design as a social activity. Their involvement in the co-designing processes described here have delivered new ways of looking at what is possible, new creative interactions, the creation of innovative tools and products for many people (not just people living with dementia) to enjoy. To evaluate the impact of these co-design projects much consideration has been given to the conversations, comments and feedback that have accompanied each co-design session. Equally important has been the observed responses by the people living with dementia to what has been going on in the co-design activities. More often than not these observations have revealed a clear willingness on the part of the people living with dementia to be involved, to take control of their own design output, and to lay claim to authorship/ownership of the creative outcomes produced. Through their demonstration of creating their designs, the people living with dementia regularly displayed independence in thinking and acting, and the importance of personal preferences. The actions, comments and feedback received in the co-design projects presented here show a strong desire of people living with dementia to be involved as well as engaging with and driving the design decisions that are needed to be taken. In all of these co-design projects, the people living with dementia have shown a strong sense of eagerness and enjoyment but also pride and esteem in their co-design work.

9 Conclusions

In the co-design projects presented in this paper, the iterative and inclusive nature of the design work leads to extended and interlinking thought processes, which in turn, results in design solutions that display the power of people living with dementia and the meaningful ways in which they can interact with and inform the world. This view presents a situation where design acts as an instigator and mediator in small and large social transactions. But more than that, the work presented in this paper has allowed the authors to access the insights, ideas and comments of people living with dementia that has resulted in designed outcomes that are directed by the people living with dementia and made accessible for the enjoyment and appreciation of other people. We believe that many of the artefacts designed in these co-design sessions have the capacity to generate financial income for their designers and as such provide alternative ways in which people living with dementia might support themselves and their families. Moreover, we believe the co-designed work presented here has the potential to change the opinions and perceptions of many in society who believe that a diagnosis of dementia represents the end of a person's creative and other abilities.

Furthermore, the personalised yet collective participation in these co-design activities supports the person living with dementia to have a better quality of life. Where the activities and contributions they make and undertake reinforces the right to active participation and citizenship, the inclusive nature of the co-design activities and resultant designed outcomes provide meaningful and relevant engagement for each individual. The co-design sessions aim to maintain the fabric of their life for as long as possible. Giving additional time to a person with dementia saves time and other valuable resources in the long run. Supporting a person to do things for themselves, rather than carrying out the task for them, maintains function and skills in their other activities of daily living. Throughout the co-design sessions described in this paper, every individual was involved in decision making, offering advice and feedback, and tasks that stimulated their motor skills. The co-design sessions have helped support the UK Government's agenda of keeping people both mentally and physically active. This approach to support continues to empower the person living with dementia to retain personal agendas within their lived experiences reaffirming capabilities and stopping people from being deemed incapable before their time. What design affords people living with dementia, in this context, is group-led and collaborative social interaction, and ultimately the production of designed outcomes that can be purchased and used by audiences beyond the natural reach of the participants. This paper clearly shows that the co-design sessions described here build self-esteem and empower people living with dementia whilst changing preconceived ideas surrounding dementia care and creating a wide range of designed outcomes that are desirable for many.

References

Cervone D (2000) Thinking about self-efficacy. Behav Modif 24(1):30–56
Cross N (2011) Design thinking: understanding how designers think and work. Bloomsbury/Berg, Oxford

Kitwood T (1997) Quality of life. In: Katz J, Peace S, Spur S (eds) Adult lives: a life course perspective. Policy Press and Open University Press, London
Muratovski G (2016) Research for designers: guide to methods and practice. Sage, London
Phillips D (2006) Quality of life. In: Katz J, Peace S, Spur S (eds) Adult lives: a life course perspective. Policy Press and Open University Press, London
Rodgers PA, Tennant A (2014) Disrupting health and social care by design. In: Proceedings of the 9th international conference on design and emotion, Bogota, Colombia, 6–10 October 2014
Scrivener S (2005) Editorial. CoDesign 1(1):1–14
Winton E, Rodgers PA (2019) Designed with me: empowering people living with dementia. Des J 22(Suppl 1):359–369

Universal Design and Child Online Protection

G. A. Giannoumis(✉) and C. Paupini

Department of Computer Science, Oslo Metropolitan University, Oslo, Norway
{gagian,cristpa}@oslomet.no

Abstract. This chapter explores the landscape of universal design and child online protection. The United Nations (UN) conceptualises child online protection as efforts to create a safe and empowering online experience for children through legal measures, technical and procedural measures, organisational structures, capacity building, and international cooperation. This chapter uses universal design as a point of departure for examining child online protection using a review of key literature and a critical analysis of select policy documents from the UN. This chapter approaches child online protection from a universal design perspective so that policymakers, information and communication technology (ICT) developers, advocates, and researchers can reframe their efforts. A universal design perspective suggests that ICT service providers must ensure that children have equal access to and use of ICT. This includes identifying and removing barriers that children experience accessing and using ICT due to, for example, their age or disability. Age-related barriers include the risks and vulnerabilities that children experience online such as exposure to harmful or dangerous content. Disability-related barriers could include, for example, the design of technical and procedural measures, such as content rating systems, that are inaccessible or unusable for children with physical, sensory, cognitive, or psychosocial disabilities.

1 Introduction

According to the United Nations (UN) Convention on the Rights of Persons with Disabilities, universal design refers to the design of, among other things, information and communication technology (ICT) to be usable by all people, to the greatest extent possible, without the need for adaptation or specialised design (UN 2006; Giannoumis and Stein 2019). Historically, universal design is rooted in conceptualisations of disability and ICT accessibility that aim to identify and remediate barriers that persons with disabilities experience accessing and using ICT (Ostroff 2011; Story 2011). However, human rights scholars have begun to re-conceptualise universal design in an effort to position universal design in relation to social equality and non-discrimination (Lid 2013; Giannoumis and Stein 2019). This reconceptualisation focuses on access to and use of ICT in relation to the breadth of human diversity. Specifically, universal design focuses on the social disadvantages that a person experiences, based on their social identities and the systems of power and privilege, which exclude and disenfranchise individuals and groups (Skjerve et al. 2016; Giannoumis and Stein 2019). According to this reconceptualisation, ICT service providers can promote universal design by, among other things, ensuring the substantive participation of diverse stakeholders in the design and development of ICT.

P. Langdon et al. (Eds.): CWUAAT 2020, *Designing for Inclusion*, pp. 13–20, 2020.
https://doi.org/10.1007/978-3-030-43865-4_2

In a separate but contiguous movement, the UN has made the protection of children online a key initiative of its cybersecurity agenda. However, despite continued efforts by the UN and national, regional, and local governments and the inter-sectoral cooperation of industry and civil society, children around the world continue to experience unsafe risks and vulnerabilities online (ITU and UNICEF 2015; ITU 2018, 2019). In addition, ICT design and development guidelines that ensure the protection of children online have yet to emerge either from industry or government.

Using the UN's conceptualisation of child online protection as a starting point (ITU 2019), this chapter examines the universal design of child online protection through a review of key literature and a critical analysis of select policy documents from the UN. This chapter approaches child online protection from a universal design perspective that takes into account ICT service providers legal and social obligations to identify and remove barriers that children experience accessing and using ICT due to, for example, their age or disability. Age-related barriers include the risks and vulnerabilities that children experience online such as exposure to harmful or dangerous content. Disability-related barriers could include, for example, the design of technical and procedural measures, such as content rating systems, that are inaccessible or unusable for children with physical, sensory, cognitive, or psychosocial disabilities. For example, a child with a disability who experiences a barrier using a content rating system may inadvertently come into contact with harmful or dangerous content.

In the past 25 years, research has produced extensive documentation of the barriers that persons with disabilities experience accessing or using ICT (Vanderheiden 1995; Brewer 2004; Blanck 2015; Lazar et al. 2015). While solutions vary, much of this literature focuses on ICT that is perceivable, operable, understandable and robust. ICT accessibility poses a particular challenge for simultaneously empowering and protecting children with disabilities. The experiences of children with cognitive and psychosocial disabilities are particularly salient as research shows a high prevalence of sexual abuse among these groups (Kvam 2000; Hershkowitz et al. 2007). This research suggests that for children with disabilities ICT must be accessible while simultaneously not increasing their vulnerability to exploitation and abuse.

However, universal design in child online protection should not be limited to considerations of age and disability. Instead, the full scope of universal design can help advocates, researchers, and policymakers better understand the unique risks and vulnerabilities that children experience online as it relates to other forms of social disadvantage such as gender and sexual orientation. In particular, from a universal design perspective, efforts to protect children online must account for the overlapping barriers that exist at the intersection of multiple forms of social disadvantage. In addition, a universal design perspective suggests that children and children with disabilities must have the opportunity to substantively participate in the design and development of ICT. By participating in the development of ICT products and services, children and children with disabilities as well as other stakeholders such as caregivers and caregivers with disabilities can provide input on the design and development process. As a result, ICT developers can use their input to consider their needs and preferences and create new universally designed ICT that embeds child protection measures in the design of ICT at an early stage.

The UN has positioned both universal design and child online protection as key considerations in the information society. By adopting universal design principles in the design and development of technical and procedural measures for child online protection, researchers, policymakers, advocates, and businesses have the opportunity to ensure that all children can safely and securely access and use ICT equally.

This chapter explores the relationship between universal design and child online protection in one specific domain, hate speech. This chapter presents five perspectives on hate speech, which focus on first anchoring hate speech as it relates to child online protection, then examining the ways in which hate speech has begun to define a generation, the emergence and diffusion of hate speech online, its regulation, and finally concludes with a comment on disablist hate speech.

2 Child Online Protection and Hate Speech

The popularisation of the Internet and World Wide Web as a means of communication has brought increased visibility to, and coordination of, extremist groups and hate-based activities (Bleich 2011). The anonymity, immediacy, and international diffusion of the Internet makes it the ideal tool for hate speech and hate-based campaigns against socially disadvantaged and marginalised groups and individuals. This chapter argues that hate speech generally refers to various forms of abuse and threats that exhibit prejudice or discrimination against disadvantaged groups. Hate speech and its analogues, cyberbullying, incitement to self-harm, and sexual predation are just some of the more severe risks and vulnerabilities that children may experience online (Del Vigna et al. 2017). Moreover, attacks can be carried out against groups of victims and can degenerate into physical violence. One form of attack, which is specific to children's protection online, is trolling. Trolling is Internet slang that refers to intentionally provoking someone into an emotional response, often by posting inflammatory, extraneous, or off-topic messages in an online community for their own amusement. The targets of "trolls" are often specific individual victims but, in some circumstances, they can target wider groups of individuals, based on disadvantaged characteristics, like race or gender (Del Vigna et al. 2017). Although experienced users might be able to face this kind of threat, most of them find themselves stuck in a mechanism that is far too strong and dangerous to handle, especially when it comes to minors.

As a result, the UN and national governments have adopted several policies and programs aimed at protection children online (ITU 2018, 2019; ITU and UNICEF 2015). The United Nations Children's Fund (UNICEF) and the UN International Telecommunication Union (ITU) have coordinated international efforts to help protect children online. For example, UNICEF (2011) has released a strategy report for dealing with the global challenge of protecting children online. The report highlights the nature and scale of abuse online, children's access to the internet, the interaction of physical and online environments, issues of risk, vulnerability, and harm, and the roles of parents and peers. It challenges the international community to develop effective international policies and other commitments, details problems faced by law enforcement, and poses a framework for responding to the need to protect children online. In a follow-up report, ITU and UNICEF (2015) outlined five key areas for protecting children online. These range from integrating child rights in organisational policies and processes, dealing with sexual abuse content and creating safer online environments, education, and using ICT for civic engagement. These key areas formed the basis for a series of general and industry-specific guidelines for mobile operators, internet service providers, content developers, online retailers, app developers, user-generated content, social media providers, broadcasting services, hardware manufacturers, operating system developers, and app stores. These reports, while integral to establishing child online protection as a global issue, have yet to acknowledge the digital risks and vulnerabilities of children with disabilities and have not fully recognised the relationship between oppressed social identities and online protection. While ITU and UNICEF (2015) does recognise the disadvantage that comes with low levels of internet access and digital literacy, it does not fully consider the role that other social identities such as gender, age, and disability play in an individual's experience of digital risk and vulnerability. In fact, despite mentioning sexual abuse over 70 times, the report does not address sexual orientation or gender once.

Starting in 2009, the ITU has released a series of guidelines for child online protection targeting children, parents and educators, industry and policymakers. The second edition of these guidelines was released in 2016 (ITU 2016). While the UN has made clear commitments to ICT accessibility for persons with disabilities (UN 2019), the very design of these guidelines means that they are not accessible to persons with disabilities.

This chapter authors found that, in an automated accessibility evaluation using Adobe Acrobat Pro DC, all the guidelines failed over half of the criteria. This does not include criteria that required a manual verification. While it is out of the scope of this chapter to test the accessibility of all of UNICEF and ITU reports on child online protection, it is worth pointing out that these reports are at the forefront of the international coordination of child online protection and their inaccessibility limits and prevents persons with disabilities accessing that information. Essentially, the inaccessibility of these reports violates the fundamental rights and obligations enshrined in the United Nations Convention on the Rights of Persons with Disabilities.

3 An Issue that Defines a Generation

Several studies found that psychological health and suicide rates among minorities groups, as well as their exclusion from society and the consequent devaluation of minority members, are linked to the public expression of hate speech (Soral et al. 2018). Hate speech uses imagery to dehumanise, and to justify exclusion and discrimination, and, in extreme cases, advocates for genocide and the elimination of groups with specific social identities. In these cases, it works by dehumanising certain groups, (and attacking the victim's dignity) and acts as a justification inciting violence and personal harm. In addition to the specific harms to individuals and groups, hate speech also shapes public opinion and condones the prejudices of people and groups in positions of power.

Initial research on hate speech focused on detection, definitions and regulations (Bleich 2011). Since the 1960s, many governments have enacted laws that penalise and criminalise hate speech and hate crimes in ways that limit the freedom of individuals to express themselves. These laws have introduced new public debates and academic research on the limits of free expression. This has focused on whether States have an obligation to limit the right to free speech in order to prevent harassment and ensure the safety of citizens. The conceptual boundaries between freedom of expression and hate speech continue to be debated. Bleich (2011) argues that hate speech violates social norms of safety and security and poses a threat to social order, similar to other forms of intergroup violence.

4 Diffusion of Hate Speech Worldwide

Shelton (1993) argued that hate speech is a growing trend among students in higher education and claimed that news media reports have steadily risen from the late 1980s to the early 1990s. Higher education institutions have responded by restricting freedom of speech and implementing policies to regulate the phenomenon. Crictics viewed these movements as a threat to the right to free speech and expression. According to these views, there is a fear that any limitation to the right to free speech will influence and justify further exceptions to free speech. Since then, numerous scholars have studied the delicate interaction between regulation of hate speech and freedom of expression, especially in the US where the First Amendment affords considerable protection to those espousing hate online (Banks 2010).

On the other hand, the Council of Europe has adopted a recommendation for how Member States approach regulating hate speech. This recommendation includes the States' responsibility in providing a legal framework for hate speech and the protection of free speech through the application of the principle of proportionality. This recommendation follows the United Nations' International Covenant on Civil and Political Rights (ICCPR), (UN 1988), that, in its 19th and 20th articles, asserts that everyone shall have the right to freedom of expression, but the exercise of this right carries with it special duties and responsibilities. It may therefore be subject to certain restrictions, for example if it contravenes the rights or reputations of others (art. 19). Along with it, any advocacy of national, racial or religious hatred that constitutes incitement to discrimination, hostility or violence shall be prohibited by law (art. 20).

5 Online Hate Speech

When it comes to the Web there are numerous issues involved in defining what constitutes hate speech and what is simply a harmless expression of a personal opinion. Merely mentioning organisations associated with hate crimes does not typically constitute hate speech. The name "Ku Klux Klan" by itself is not hateful, as it may appear in historical articles, legal documents, or other legitimate communication. Even an endorsement of the organisation does not constitute a verbal attack on another group (Warner and Hirschberg 2012). Defining and individuating hate speech online has been a focus of academic research in the last ten years. Recently scholars have developed lexicon-based methodologies and crawling systems, which included a hate speech classifier for detecting violent discussions on the Web (Del Vigna et al. 2017). However, the technology industry remains at the forefront in monitoring and removing hate speech (Perrigo 2020).

6 Concluding Remarks on Ablist Hate Speech

The links between universal design, child online protection and the experiences of children with disabilities with online hate speech are complex. This article has set up a potential premise for connecting universal design and child online protection. Universal design provides a framework for ensuring access to ICT for everyone. This includes ensuring access to the web for children with disabilities. However, the UN recognises that children with disabilities are a specialised group whose rights are distinct from the larger population of persons with disabilities. This is due, in part, to the vulnerability of children with disabilities to exploitation and abuse. Although access to the web can empower children with disabilities to participate in society, it also opens up a new channel for exploitation and abuse. Therefore, policies and programs must recognise the complex challenges for ensuring access to the web for children with disabilities while at the same time protecting them from hate speech and other forms of online violence. For example, ICT tools, awareness raising information, and other online protection efforts must be accessible for persons with disabilities generally and must specifically recognise the needs of children with disabilities.

Although academic interest has been growing around hate speech, little research has been conducted about hate speech in relation to persons with disability (Olsen et al. 2016). Internet trolls typically target members of disadvantaged groups, but it is very rare that disability is recognised as one of these groups. Research has shown that in an 'offline' context, persons with disabilities are more likely to face harassment and hate than persons without disabilities (Emerson 2014) and that this victimisation is probably linked with health conditions or stigma. Reported motivations for harassment ranged from hate, jealousy, stigma, stereotypes (of life not worth living), and accusations of fraud in cases of invisible impairments (Quarmby 2012, 2015). The popularisation of the Internet have made it possible to exploit ICT channels, virtual environments, and the anonymity of offenders. This has exposed persons with disabilities to online hate speech and other offences (Wells and Mitchell 2014).

Despite active research that has explored numerous aspects and issues related to hate speech, few scholars have analysed the problem in relation to persons with disability. At the time of writing this chapter only four research papers specifically engage with the topic of ablist online hate speech. In two papers, Burnap and Williams (2015, 2016) identify the use of 'othering' language on Twitter, based on race, disability and sexual orientation. In this case persons with disabilities are recognised as a discriminated minority group, but the aim of the research is to develop a machine classification system to code tweets and individuate hate speech expressions. As such, it does not focus on laws and policies that can regulate online hate speech. In a third paper, Alhaboby et al. (2016) use an online survey to explore the personal impacts of disability-related cyber-hate and cyber-harassment, without connecting this to wider discourses surrounding hate speech. In the fourth and most recent paper, Leah Burch explores how the meta-narrative of disability as a drain on the so-called "hard working taxpayers" is articulated in the online bulletin board, Reddit, and the author shows how disablist hate speech may emerge as an attempt to secure one's sense of self during austere times.

This chapter hopes to inform future research by providing a justification for examining the mechanisms that trigger hate speech online and how persons with disabilities experience it. It suggests that research could usefully examine the extent that social networks policies cover ablist hate speech and their actions to prevent it. It is necessary to fill this gap because the 'harms' of hate are not solely experienced within the realm of an individual. Instead, harms transgress boundaries, moving between personal, social and cultural spaces. It seems the case, however, that disablist hate speech has become normalised to the point that its harms are not recognised (Burch 2018).

References

Alhaboby ZA, al-Khateeb HM, Barnes J, Short E (2016) The language is disgusting and they refer to my disability: the cyberharassment of disabled people. Disabil Soc 31(8):1138–1143

Banks J (2010) Regulating hate speech online. Int Rev Law Comput Technol 24(3):233–239

Blanck P (2015) eQuality: web accessibility by people with cognitive disabilities. J Inf 3(2):75–91

Bleich E (2011) The rise of hate speech and hate crime laws in liberal democracies. J Ethn Migr Stud 37(6):917–934

Brewer J (2004) Web accessibility highlights and trends. In: Proceedings of the 2004 international cross-disciplinary workshop on web accessibility (W4A), New York, NY, US, 17–22 May 2004

Burch L (2018) You are a parasite on the productive classes: online disablist hate speech in austere times. Disabil Soc 33(3):392–415

Burnap P, Williams ML (2015) Cyber hate speech on Twitter: an application of machine classification and statistical modeling for policy and decision making. Policy Internet 7(2):223–242

Burnap P, Williams ML (2016) Us and them: identifying cyber hate on Twitter across multiple protected characteristics. EPJ Data Sci 5(1):11

Del Vigna F, Cimino A, Dell'Orletta F, Petrocchi M, Tesconi M (2017) Hate me, hate me not: hate speech detection on facebook. In: Paper presented at the proceedings of the first Italian conference on cybersecurity (ITASEC 2017), Venice, Italy, 17–20 January 2017

Dell'Orletta F, Venturi G, Cimino A, Montemagni S (2014) T2k^2: a system for automatically extracting and organizing knowledge from texts. In: Proceedings of the 9th international conference on language resources and evaluation (LREC 2014), Reykjavik, Iceland, 26–31 May 2014

Emerson E (2014) Disability, hate crime and violence. Disabil Soc 29(3):495–496

Giannoumis GA, Stein M (2019) Conceptualizing universal design for the information society through a universal human rights lens. Int Hum Rights Law Rev 8(1):38–66

Hershkowitz I, Lamb ME, Horowitz D (2007) Victimization of children with disabilities. Am J Orthopsychiatry 77(4):629–635

ITU (2016) Guidelines. www.itu.int/en/cop/Pages/guidelines.aspx. Accessed 16 Jan 2020

ITU (2018) Presentations from the ITU Regional Workshop for Europe and CIS on Cybersecurity and Child Online Protection. www.itu.int/en/ITU-D/Regional-Presence/CIS/Pages/EVENTS/2018/04_Odessa/04_Odessa_Presentations.aspx. Accessed 16 Jan 2020

ITU (2019) About the child online protection initiative. www.itu.int/en/cop/Pages/about_cop.aspx. Accessed 16 Jan 2020

ITU and UNICEF (2015) Guidelines for industry on child online protection. The International Telecommunication Union (ITU) and UNICE. www.unicef.org/csr/files/COP_Guidelines_English.pdf. Accessed 16 Jan 2020

Kvam MH (2000) Is sexual abuse of children with disabilities disclosed? A retrospective analysis of child disability and the likelihood of sexual abuse among those attending Norwegian hospitals. Child Abuse Negl 24(8):1073–1084

Lazar J, Goldstein DF, Taylor A (2015) Ensuring digital accessibility through process and policy. Morgan Kaufmann/Elsevier Publishers, Waltham

Lid IM (2013) Developing the theoretical content in universal design. Scand J Disabil Res 15(3):203–215

Olsen T, Vedeler J, Eriksen J, Elvegård K (2016) Hatytringer. Resultater fra en studie av funksjonshemmedes erfaringer. Nordlandsforskning 6/16, Bodø, Norway

Ostroff E (2011) Universal design: an evolving paradigm. In: Smith KH, Preiser WFE (eds) Universal design handbook. McGraw-Hill, New York

Perrigo B (2020) Facebook says it's removing more hate speech than ever before. But there's a catch. time.com/5739688/facebook-hate-speech-languages/. Accessed 15 Jan 2020

Quarmby K (2012) Media reporting and disability hate crime. In: Roulstone A, Mason-Bish H (eds) Disability, hate crime and violence. Routledge, Abingdon

Quarmby K (2015) Disability hate crime motivation survey–results. katharinequarmby.wordpress.com/. Accessed 16 Jan 2020

Shelton MW (1993) Hateful help – a practical look at the issue of hate speech. In: Paper presented at the annual meeting of the speech communication association, Miami, FL, US. files.eric.ed.gov/fulltext/ED367041.pdf. Accessed 16 Jan 2020

Skjerve R, Giannoumis GA, Naseem S (2016) An intersectional perspective on web accessibility. In: Langdon PM et al (eds) Designing around people. Springer, Cham

Soral W, Bilewicz M, Winiewski M (2018) Exposure to hate speech increases prejudice through desensitization. Aggressive Behav 44(2):136–146

Story MF (2011) The principles of universal design. In: Smith KH, Preiser WFE (eds) Universal design handbook. McGraw-Hill, New York

UN (1988) The International Bill of Human Rights: Universal Declaration of Human Rights: International Covenant on Economic, Social and Cultural Rights: International Covenant on Civil and Political Rights and Optional Protocol. United Nations, New York, NY, US

UN (2006) Convention on the Rights of Persons with Disabilities and Optional Protocol (9789211302615921 1302617). https://www.un.org/development/desa/disabilities/convention-on-the-rights-of-persons-with-disabilities.html. Accessed 16 Jan 2020

UN (2019) United Nations disability inclusion strategy. www.un.org/en/events/disabilitiesday/assets/pdf/UN-Disability-Inclusion-Strategy.pdf. Accessed 16 Jan 2020

UNICEF (2011) Child safety online. Global challenges and strategies. Unisef Innocenti Research Centre. www.unicef-irc.org/publications/pdf/ict_eng.pdf. Accessed 16 Jan 2020

Vanderheiden G (1995) Design of HTML (mosaic) pages to increase their accessibility to users with disabilities strategies for today and tomorrow version 1.0. Trace R& D Center, University of Wisconsin, Madison, WI, US. https://perma.cc/7ME-QUNC. Accessed 16 Jan 2020

Warner W, Hirschberg J (2012) Detecting hate speech on the world wide web. In: Proceedings of the 2nd workshop on language in social media, Montréal, Canada, 7 June 2012

Wells M, Mitchell KJ (2014) Patterns of internet use and risk of online victimization for youth with and without disabilities. J Spec Educ 48(3):204–213

Designing Inclusive Assistive and Rehabilitation Systems

Sleepwear for Breast Cancer Survivors: Enacting Inclusion Through Feminine Identity and Attachments

S. Tullio-Pow[1](✉), K. Schaefer[1], J. Nyhof-Young[2], and M. Strickfaden[3]

[1] School of Fashion, Ryerson University, Toronto, ON, Canada
{stullio,kirsten.schaefer}@ryerson.ca
[2] Department of Family and Community Medicine, University of Toronto, Toronto, ON, Canada
joyce.nyhof-young@uhn.ca
[3] Department of Human Ecology, University of Alberta, Edmonton, AB, Canada
megan.strickfaden@ualberta.ca

Abstract. Clothing is an integral part of material culture. It does more than simply cover and protect the body. This chapter reports findings of a study on women's perceptions of sleepwear specifically designed for their unique body forms after breast cancer surgery (mastectomy or lumpectomy). Women's perceptions are naturally linked to societal ideals of beauty and women's identities are related to body forms and clothing silhouettes. Wardrobes typically include different types of sleepwear that usually fall into three categories: commodity sleepwear, loungewear, and lingerie. Our research methodology used a participatory, user-centred framework that included email interviews with 37 women with asymmetrical or missing breasts after cancer surgery who were given specially designed sleepwear for field-testing. After a 3-month period, questions about hypothetical loss of the clothing prompted participant responses that revealed strong and weak attachments to the sleepwear and how it is used to re-script feminine identities. The results are explored to better understand self-identity and women's identities in relation to others. Our study reveals how clothing aids people in everyday and natural human performances that reinforce societal narratives.

1 Introduction

Clothing is an integral part of material culture. It does more than simply cover and protect the body, as is evidenced by many papers and books about people's complex relationships with their clothes (e.g., Miller 2005; Woodward 2007; Twigg 2013). Furthermore, notions of beauty, being beautiful by wearing clothing, and the creation of women's identities through clothing are integral to people's positions, relationships and perceptions within society. For example, a woman's identity as defined through society often relates to the aesthetics of femininity which "include having, or at least appearing to have, two full breasts" (Spence 2001, p. 175).

Women's breasts also hold cultural significance; they are "glorified and equated with femininity, sexual attractiveness and nurturing behavior" (Kaiser 1990, p. 134). Given the cultural importance of breasts in our society, most women with mastectomies

P. Langdon et al. (Eds.): CWUAAT 2020, *Designing for Inclusion*, pp. 23–34, 2020.
https://doi.org/10.1007/978-3-030-43865-4_3

or lumpectomies following breast cancer surgery wear a prosthesis. The practice of wearing a prosthesis allows women to maintain the illusion of a traditional female form and avoid stigma, or what Goffman (1963) describes as "passing" in society. Women who choose to conceal the results of their breast cancer surgery constantly manage the "tension generated during social contacts…. To display or not to display; to tell or not to tell; to let on or not; to lie or not to lie; and in each case, to whom, how, when and where" (Goffman 1963, p. 42).

Successfully carrying out the illusion of having symmetrical breasts requires the "right clothing," as the opacity of the fabric, cut of the neckline, the depth of the armhole and the brassiere itself may all potentially expose and thus stigmatise a woman. As evidenced through extensive literature summaries, a multitude of studies query women's perceptions of clothing. Women who have survived breast cancer have been the focus of research to determine the stigma of clothing post-mastectomy (Feather et al. 1989) and their needs related to breast prostheses, mastectomy bras and lymphedema sleeves (LaBat et al. 2017), brassieres for exercising (Gho et al. 2014) as well as their experiences with their changed bodies (Brunet et al. 2013). Although Winkler (1977) highlighted clothing challenges inherent in nightgowns, bathing suits and evening gowns, we could find no literature exploring women's perceptions about clothing following a major change in body form such as breast cancer. Furthermore, it is well known that most women have a wide variety of clothing in their closets and dresser drawers, yet little to no research exists within the fashion domain of sleepwear. Research on clothing for unique body forms is also scant and often focuses on designing for a specific disability and context (e.g., job interviews and outdoor clothing) rather than investigating women's perceptions and reflections on how they are attached to clothing.

Consequently, this study looks into women's perceptions of sleepwear that is designed for their unique body forms after breast cancer surgery. Effectively concealing a missing breast in daywear is less problematic than doing so in more revealing sleepwear silhouettes due to fabrics and fit that are naturally designed to be somewhat revealing. Women's wardrobes typically include different types of sleepwear, much of which is of the basic commodity variety. Commodity sleepwear includes cotton or flannel nightgowns, pajamas and bath robes that are often worn around the house and sometimes in bed. Some of their sleepwear will be loungewear, and perhaps a few pieces will be categorised as lingerie. Loungewear comprises the types of clothes some women change into early in the evening when relaxing. Loungewear is comfortable and is sometimes slept in but also may be worn in the company of others because of its fabric and styling. While a woman might feel uncomfortable if guests dropped by unexpectedly when she was dressed in commodity sleepwear, she would feel appropriate in the company of close friends or family in loungewear. The third category of sleepwear is lingerie, which has another purpose altogether: sending the message of romance to a partner. Lingerie is typically made from lace, silky and/or sheer fabrics, in styles that are more revealing and aimed toward creating an atmosphere of intimacy. Lingerie may indeed be slept in but it is rarely worn in the company of anyone other than a lover as a suggestion of intimacy. While commodity sleepwear and loungewear pose fewer problems for women who have unique body forms, lingerie is an entirely different matter. With commodity sleepwear and loungewear worn in the comfort and privacy of their homes, many women would remove their brassiere and the prosthesis contained within it, which creates a problem: Without the brassiere as an essential undergarment to contain a prosthesis, it is impossible for women to create the illusion of ideal beauty, and this can negatively impact self-esteem, body image and sexual quality of life (Emilee et al. 2010).

This chapter brings together theories on identity and attachment with the aim of understanding women's deep and meaningful relationships with clothing. To begin we elaborate upon these theories as they relate to clothing. This is followed by describing our study methodology, as well as the novel sleepwear that was provided to our participants—women who had breast cancer surgery. We continue with our findings that illustrate how attachments are indicators of identity and how feminine identities can be re-scripted through clothing.

2 Identity and Attachment to Clothing

It is well known among scholars who study clothing that it communicates a great deal of information about the self: age, gender, occupation, socioeconomic status, class, as well as mood and personality (e.g. Ryan 1966). Clothing and identity are closely linked (Stone 1962), with identity defined here as "the self-in-context—a self that is embedded in social relations and situations" (Kaiser 1990, p. 96). The clothing–identity link is exemplified in research such as Partington's (2014) study of class and clothing. Elaborating upon identity, Davis (1992) indicates that social identities do not remain the same throughout a person's life because identity is constantly in flux, "in production" (Hall 1996, p. 6), "performative" (Partington 2014, p. 8) and in active participation "in the development of new styles of dress and the development of their own identities" (Partington 2014, pp. 7–8). This performance of identity is evident when examining the changed identities of breast cancer survivors, as "the post-diagnosis and post-operative self can never be what it was before breast cancer" (Spence 2001, p. 176). Active participation is demonstrated each day when women wear a prosthesis or choose clothing that creates the illusion of a traditional silhouette, rather than emphasising their unique forms created through surgery.

Attachment through material possessions, including attachment to clothing, is defined as the relationship between a person and material objects (Kleine and Baker 2004). Norman (2005) discusses the impact of designed objects on people, indicating that objects are interpreted by people on visceral, behavioural and reflective ways that result in multifaceted levels of attraction. Norman elaborates upon person–object attachments, suggesting that specific regions of the brain are responsible for different processes and decisions. He argues that visceral attachments are rapid and automatic, and often based on physical appearances that result in immediate judgments. People may ask questions that indicate their attachments when choosing clothing, such as "Is this pretty or ugly?" or "Is it me or not me?" (Kleine et al. 1995). Norman (2005) describes behavioural attachments as being linked to less conscious reasoning and related to use and performance, which include an object's function, understandability, usability and physical feel. Finally, Norman describes reflective attachments as being related to people's self-image, the meaning of the product and the signal it sends to others. When considering attachments in this complex way, it is clear that people become attached to objects such as clothing in various ways and with various intensities. For instance, some researchers believe that feelings of attachment to objects manifest differently for each person and can be described as being on a continuum from weak to strong (Kleine et al. 1995). Thus, the manner in which and level that an object connects with an individual will influence the intensity of attachment. This relationship with material objects is inherently linked to a person's identity because individuals extend themselves into (and through) their personal possessions (Csikszentmihalyi and Rochberg-Halton 1981; Belk 1988). Furthermore, claims have been made that attachment relative to taste in clothing "needs to be understood as the transformative production of new identities that are 'temporary attachments to subjective positions'" (Partington 2014, p. 15).

To more fully appreciate the perceptions of women who have had surgery for breast cancer and the relationship they have with their clothes, it is important to understand the context and repertoire of attachments associated with identity, which includes recognising the ways that people perform in front of different audiences (Tseëlon 1995). Ryan (1966) defines the "somatic self" as the physical attributes of the body and the "social self" as the way a person interacts with another person or a group. Body image is delineated as "the picture individuals have in their minds about how they look to others" whereas body cathexis may be described as the level of satisfaction one has about their body (Horn and Gurel 1981). Body cathexis relates to self-esteem, which Kaiser (1990) portrays as a person's confidence and sense of worth. "Because body parts are normally central to conceptions of self, the loss of body parts is tantamount to losing one's identity and one's very being" (Belk 1988, p. 157). Thus, it is difficult to fully appreciate the impact of the loss of a breast—a part of the body that is so integrated with cultural ideals of beauty and femininity—on the multiple facets of a woman's self-identity and the subsequent rupture of attachment to clothing. Although research shows that women who survive breast cancer must reconstruct themselves "both mentally and physically," this cannot be accomplished with a prosthesis and clothing alone (Spence 2001). Like Belk (1988), we believe that clothing and other possessions can help women manage, re-script, perform and realise their ongoing self-identities.

3 Design Research and Methodology

The research reported in this chapter is the last phase of an ongoing series of design research completed by a leading Canadian cancer hospital and university School of Fashion. They collaborated to investigate the clothing challenges of women with unique body forms, specifically women who had undergone breast surgery, in order to design clothing using a participatory, user-centred design framework (Martin and Hanington 2012). Active involvement of our participants in the design process facilitated the sharing of opinions and thus promoted deep understanding. Phase I of this research explored women's post-mastectomy sleepwear concerns and preferences through focus group interviews and surveys ($n = 18$). Findings included the physical and emotional impact of mastectomy on women, as well as clothing needs and preferences related to cost, colour, comfort and cut (Tullio-Pow et al. 2011a). In Phase II, sleepwear designs were developed, called *Sweetdreams*; see Fig. 1 (Tullio-Pow et al. 2011b). In Phase III, sleepwear designs were prototyped, wear tested on a fit model, revised and manufactured for field-testing.

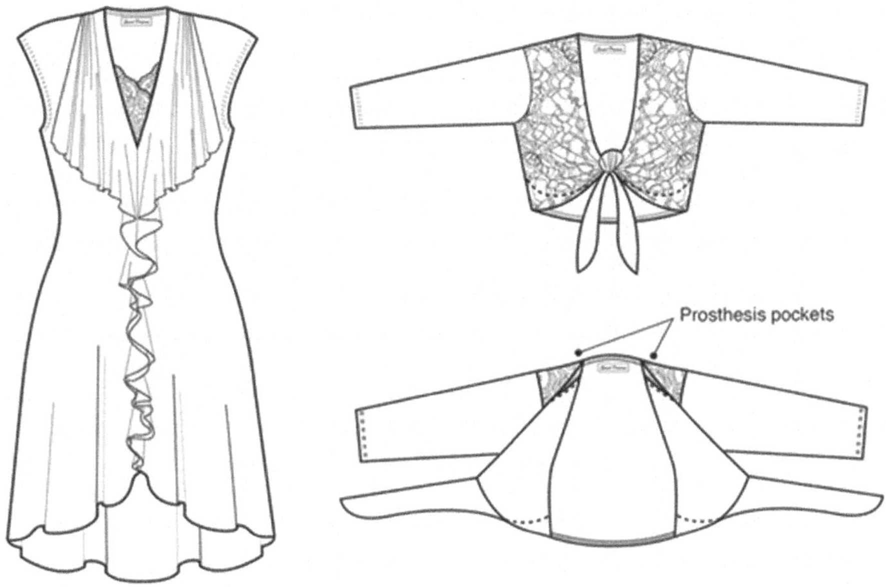

Fig. 1. Sleepwear including a nightgown and jacket set

In conjunction with our participatory design framework, the *Sweetdreams* sleepwear was designed based on women's preferences, desires and needs that included: a traditional symmetrical silhouette, placement of seams in relation to scars, and consideration of the discomfort caused by hot flashes, a common side effect of cancer treatment (Tullio-Pow et al. 2011a). Designing the nightgown and jacket set in collaboration with women who wished to have options for sleepwear, in particular loungewear and lingerie, incorporated inclusive design principles (Story 2001) and used Lamb and Kallal's (1992) FEA model that identifies clothing as having functional, expressive and aesthetic attributes. Our design outcome embodies fit and comfort (functional), considers a woman's feelings of modesty and appearance (expressive) and incorporates attractive detailing, feminine styling and fabrics in contemporary colours (aesthetics).

The sleepwear set is cut from a rayon (from bamboo) and cotton blend, jersey knit fabric that has a soft hand, superior absorbency and wicking abilities, all meant to enhance the wearer's comfort by minimising the effects of hot flashes. Lace is the secondary material used as a small segment in the neckline of the nightgown camisole and as an overlay on the front of the jacket to provide added support to the delicate jersey knit fabric.

The nightgown silhouette is semi-fitted to the waist, flaring out to a length just below the back of the knee. Styling includes a V-neck with a draped collar; the proportion is engineered to provide fullness over the bust area to camouflage breast asymmetry. The inside seam of the V-neckline is stabilised with narrow clear elastic to prevent stretching. The base of the collar transforms into a cascading ruffle that is integrated into the centre front seam, decreasing in width from neckline to hem. A V-neck camisole is a layer attached to the front inside of the nightgown, extending to the waistline. During garment assembly, the back and front side seams are stitched so as to completely enclose the seams within the front camisole panel, eliminating rough edges that might irritate tender scars and sensitive skin. Two sections of soft, knitted lace are positioned to overlap one another at the base of the V-neck so as to conceal cleavage unevenness, scars and radiation tattoos. A small cap sleeve covers the shoulder, and the armhole is cut with consideration to scars in the armpit area where lymph nodes may have been removed. Seams along the back neck and armhole are flat locked; this stitch type completely encloses the raw edge of the seam within the stitching on the side of the garment next to the body and forms two rows of topstitching on the outer side of the garment. Label, care content and size tags are located at the back neck. The hem is tulip shaped, slightly shorter in the front than in the back. The side seams are serged, a stitch formation that maintains the inherent stretch of the knit fabric and encloses the raw edges of the seams within the stitches. The hem edges, and those along the collar and ruffle, are finished with fine, baby-lock seams.

The jacket is a semi-fitted bolero style, the centre back proportioned just above the waist with a hemline that curved upward to a centre front tie. The ¾-length sleeve is cut slightly more generously than a traditional sleeve to accommodate increased arm girth due to lymphedema (a chronic condition that may impact women after breast cancer treatment). The shoulder seam allowance includes a length of India-tape to prevent stretching. All seam layers at the shoulder are enclosed within the front jacket panel to eliminate any potentially rough seam edges. Prosthesis pockets on the right and left side of the jacket are accessible through each corresponding side of the inside front neckline. The front panels utilise an overlay of firm, structured, net lace in order to stabilise and minimise the stretch of the jersey knit when a prosthesis is inserted. An arc of topstitching through all layers of the front jacket panel forms a pocket to hold the prosthesis in place. The back neck is flat-lock stitched and includes a length of narrow, clear elastic to limit excessive stretch through wear. A label, care content and size tag are located at the centre back neck. The sleeves are serged to the jacket armhole, and the seam allowance is pressed into the sleeve. The jacket and sleeve hems are also finished with flat-lock stitching. All layers of the jacket side seam are enclosed within the front panel for a clean finish inside.

The sleepwear design was created for and with women who had undergone a significant change in their body form due to breast cancer surgery. This chapter focuses on the experiences of women who wore and reflected upon the sleepwear. Their feedback is examined to gain a deeper understanding of their perceptions about clothing and identity. A group of 37 women who had undergone breast cancer surgery responded to our recruitment email announcement in a breast prosthesis manufacturer's blog and agreed to field test our specially designed sleepwear set (value $125 CAD) for a nominal fee ($20 CAD) to cover shipping and handling. After approximately 3 weeks, participants were contacted to set up a mutually agreeable time to participate in an audio-recorded phone interview to determine satisfaction with garment fit and functionality, feelings while wearing the sleepwear, opinions about styling, preferences regarding alternate fabrics (based on swatches provided) and lastly durability during laundering and care.

This chapter reports on the next stage of investigation. After a cooling-off period of 3 months, the group was emailed three additional follow-up questions to further query their attachments to the sleepwear and to understand how the sleepwear related to their ongoing performance of self-identity. The women were asked if they were still wearing the sleepwear, and if so, how frequently. We also asked about their current perceptions of the design. Questions about hypothetical loss (Martin and Hanington 2012) were used to further prompt participants' responses. We asked: The sleepwear was not part of your wardrobe four months ago; now that it is, what role does it play in your life? Consider how you might feel if this sleepwear was lost (e.g., your luggage was lost by an airline when returning from a trip) or if your sleepwear was damaged (e.g., laundered with bleach by accident).

A total of 37 women responded. Email responses from each participant were copied verbatim into one document for analysis. Individual responses were then cross-referenced to demographic information in order to track whether participants' perceptions were unique to their stage of post-surgery rehabilitation. Most women were between the ages of 51 and 70 (n = 23). All had undergone lumpectomy or mastectomy surgery, and three had breast reconstruction. Some of the women had finished treatment and come to terms with their new bodies because they had been diagnosed with breast cancer a decade or more ago (n = 6). Many had passed the 5-year survivor threshold (n = 13); others were approaching this benchmark (n = 6), while some women were relatively naïve to their new bodies, given they were less than 2 years post-treatment (n = 6). Most of the women were married/living with a partner (n = 22); several had children living at home (n = 5) and some lived alone (n = 9). The first author conducted descriptive thematic analysis of the women's responses, systematically searching for levels of attachment and how participants articulated their sense of self when wearing the sleepwear. Categories were reviewed and discussed with the senior author to confirm analytic trustworthiness, and the broader team confirmed interpretations.

The sleepwear set designed with and for women who had undergone breast cancer surgery was integral to our research goal of understanding these women's relationship with sleepwear before and after surgery. The clothing design research provided our participants with an opportunity to compare their past and present selves and their past and present sleepwear. This comparison in turn allowed for deeper explorations into person–object attachments and the multiple facets of a person's self-identity.

4 Attachments as Indicators of Identity

Attachments to objects, whether strong or weak, are indicators of individuals' self-identities and their identities in relation to other people. Even though clothing is often considered something that displays people to one another, Tseëlon (1995) maintains that the self is also an audience—"how one feels about oneself even when nobody is looking" draws "a parallel between inner feeling and appearance". As such, a strong attachment means that people can work with or use an object towards a greater purpose such as creating meaning for themselves or with others. Many of the women in our study referenced our sleepwear as something *comfortable* and *special to wear* that made them *look attractive*. When interpreted, these seemingly simple statements tell us about the values of these women. They desire feelings of well-being to maintain or re/create their feminine identities.

Many well-articulated statements by these women suggest strong attachments. One woman's words are particularly telling:

> *I would be very upset if something happened to my post-mastectomy sleepwear as I wear it all the time, sometimes don't take it off during the day. I find it very comfortable. It's like an old pair of socks that you really love and don't want to give them up even though they have holes and your big toe is totally sticking out. That's the best example of how much I love this sleepwear.* (TK)

Other examples of strong attachments to the sleepwear are evidenced through some of the women's comments about how they missed their sleepwear when it was being laundered, cared for it carefully during laundering, and preserved it by wearing it only on special occasions. One woman said, "I take good care of my clothing, so it has washed beautifully. I have dried it by hanging it outside as I do with most of my clothing" (DL). Another said,

> *I feel really good in it…I only use it on special occasions and have not washed it that much. I find it very comfortable but do not want to wear it out by wearing it while I am by myself.* (HM)

A powerful statement made by one woman shows a particularly strong attachment to the sleepwear. She invested time in modifying her nightgown and jacket:

> *With regards to the pockets in the jacket, they need to be raised because otherwise the prosthesis sits far too low on the chest, I just sewed a horizontal seam and it worked perfectly. The only other concern that I had was the front of the nightgown was too short for my needs. If I was just wearing it to bed it would be fine, but to wear it with company present or grandkids, it was a little immodest. I solved that problem by sewing a lined lace panel in the front and that evened the hemline for me. I also ended up purchasing another black soft cotton nightgown, ankle length and I wear the jacket with that nightgown when my [Sweetdreams] nightgown is in the wash.* (MSG)

These examples of strong attachments illustrate how a seemingly simple nightgown is a significant object, or perhaps even an actor, in performing self-identities and building social relationships. However, some of the women in our study spoke of weaker attachments. It is interesting to explore how these relate to the women's identities.

Some women showed weak attachments to the sleepwear, even though they appreciated receiving a free nightgown designed with their unique needs in mind. One woman stated openly that she "does not get attached to very many items of clothing" (HP). Another explained her lack of attachment with reasons such as the colour and cost of the sleepwear. Other women noted that they might have appreciated the sleepwear more if it were a gift. In one woman's words, "if someone had thought enough to purchase it for me, then I might feel more sentimental about it" (HJ). These women's perceptions of the sleepwear highlight the importance of the look and cost of clothing, as well as how people relate to objects they acquire as gifts. According to Norman (2005), colour is an object attribute that influences visceral decision-making and is highly subjective. It is interesting to note that being partial to a particular colour for daywear may not translate to sleepwear. Much of commodity sleepwear seems to be manufactured in pastel colours or jewel tones and lingerie sometimes comes in black. The nightgown and jacket in this study can be used in a variety of ways; for example, as commodity sleepwear or lingerie. This means that its colour needs to reflect both these categories. The cost of sleepwear is relative to many factors such as the women's buying habits and socioeconomic status. This can also be understood through Norman's description of reflective decision-making whereby people qualify the benefits of the sleepwear in comparison to cost. In respect to objects that are given as gifts, Belk (1988) indicates how gifts offer stronger attachments because a "gift continues to be associated with the giver". These women's statements about their weak attachments to sleepwear tell us how their identities are linked to more than just themselves. The women's statements are stories about how they define beauty and incorporate it into their lives (colour, style), their socioeconomic position in society (cost) and how they create meaning through and with objects (associating them with other people).

5 Re-scripting Feminine Identities

If clothing is an actor in the ongoing performance of identity creation, then clothing has the potential to re-script feminine identities. What appears at first to be a weak attachment between one woman and her sleepwear is a striking illustration of how one woman's identity transitioned from one phase of healing to another. She talks about her sleepwear:

> *It has become part of the rotation of sleepwear with no more or no less importance than other things I wear. I have become more comfortable with the mastectomy, so it has less importance that I thought it might. At the beginning (immediately after surgery) I was always looking for clothes to hide it...now that isn't as important to me.* (AM)

This particular woman was diagnosed with breast cancer less than 6 months prior. She talks about a distinct shift in her identity from wishing to pass as being the same to accepting that she now has a unique body form. One wonders how that identity shift will continue as her survivorship journey evolves over time. This woman's transition is a tangible example of her active participation in performing her identity through clothing. Her personal journey naturally impacts her clothing choices and her relationships with other people.

Spence (2001) discusses her personal experience with breast cancer and explains how "women are peculiarly sensitive to 'the gaze' of others, and are used to considering themselves through the eyes of the observer". As such, it is not surprising that other women in our study openly expressed feeling empowered by the symbolic powers imbued within their sleepwear. For example, one woman said "I get compliments from my spouse" and another elaborated on how the sleepwear acts as a transformational object that aids in creating intimate connections with her husband:

This outfit plays a special role in my life and I would miss it greatly if it were lost. The outfit makes me feel much more feminine. I wear it during special times with my husband... an evening to ourselves, a candlelight dinner, a special bottle of wine. It almost makes the past seven years melt away and I forget the insults that my body has endured. My husband reacts to it because I am in a different place when I wear it. Funny to say that a mere piece of clothing can help a relationship. (CK)

The sleepwear not only had apparent meaning in intimate relationships but also provoked a sense of physical comfort related to maintaining modesty and an appropriate sense of decorum around other people. Commonly, the women in our study mentioned that they felt they had something special to take when travelling, especially because they knew they would be in the company of other people. One woman said,

I've had a number of house guests in the past few months, as well as sleepovers with grandchildren. I love this nightgown because I can wear it around the house and not worry about getting dressed first thing in the morning. (MSG)

Another said,

*We are going to Vancouver for Christmas to be with our son and I am so looking forward to not having to get dressed in street clothes early in the [*morning*] but just lounge around in my sleepwear.* (JMZ)

These statements about how the sleepwear communicates with others illustrates how clothing can act as mediating devices between or among people. Clearly a nightgown and jacket are not just pieces of cloth covering body parts: They aid people in everyday and natural human performances that reinforce societal narratives, such as how to feel and act sexily and how to interact with family members in appropriate ways. That is, when a woman feels comfortable in her own body, the result is a better connection with others. Therefore, we believe that the symbolic aspects of garments are valued as devices to enable and support what the wearer wishes to achieve socially.

6 Conclusion

Feminine identities have been associated with the curves of the female body for many decades and are naturally linked to accentuated forms such as the bust and bottom. In our society, millions of dollars, pounds and euros are spent each year on plastic surgery to enhance what are defined as "feminine curves." The mere concept of "the bust" implies a natural symmetry between a woman's two breasts, even when the majority of women are naturally asymmetrical. These societal narratives play deeply into women's perceptions of beauty and their identities relating to body forms and clothing silhouettes.

Throughout our discussions and email interviews with the women who had breast cancer surgery and wore sleepwear specially designed for them, we deepened our understanding of how clothing is used to perform identity and enact inclusion—inclusion in family activities, social gatherings in the home and intimate romantic interludes. These performances are about women's self-identities and how they create social relationships with others. The attachments that people create with objects comprise a deeply complex process among connections, disconnections and how clothes act to communicate messages to other people in ways similar to language (McCracken 1988). Those attachments are "magic vessels" of meaning (Belk 1991). The women in our study tell us what it is like to be breast cancer survivors with mastectomies and lumpectomies, and about the strong attachments, weak attachments, special moments or memories, transformations and connections with people, all mediated through a nightgown designed specifically for their altered body habitus. Most importantly, however, as emphasised by other material culture scholars, we can begin to model generalisable person–object relationships through the specific voices and experiences of women.

References

Belk R (1988) Possessions and the extended self. J Consum Res 15:139–168

Belk R (1991) Possessions and the sense of past. In: Belk RW (ed) Highways and buyways: naturalistic research from the consumer behavior odyssey. Association for Consumer Research, Provo

Brunet J, Sabiston CM, Burke S (2013) Surviving breast cancer: women's experiences with their changed bodies. Body Image 10:344–351

Csikszentmihalyi M, Rochberg-Halton E (1981) The meaning of things. Cambridge University Press, New York

Davis F (1992) Fashion, culture, and identity. University of Chicago Press, Chicago

Emilee G, Ussher JM, Perz J (2010) Sexuality after breast cancer: a review. Maturitas 66:397–407

Feather BL, Rucker M, Kaiser SB (1989) Social concerns of post-mastectomy women: stigmata and clothing. Home Econ Res J 17:289–299

Gho SA, Munro BJ, Jones SC, Steele JR (2014) Evidence-based recommendations for building better bras for women treated for breast cancer. Ergonomics 57:774–786

Goffman E (1963) Stigma. Simon & Schuster, New York

Hall S (1996) Introduction: who needs "identity"? In: Hall S, du Gay P (eds) Questions of cultural identity. Sage, London

Horn M, Gurel L (1981) The second skin, 3rd edn. Houghton-Mifflin, Boston

Kaiser S (1990) The social psychology of clothing: symbolic appearances in context, 2nd edn. Macmillan, New York

Kleine S, Baker S (2004) An integrative review of material possession attachment. Acad Mark Sci Rev 8:1–35

Kleine S, Kleine R, Allen C (1995) How is a possession "me" or "not me"? Characterizing types and an antecedent of material possession attachment. J Consum Res 22:327–343

LaBat KL, Ryan KS, Sanden-Will S (2017) Breast cancer survivors' wearable product needs and wants: a challenge to designers. Int J Fash Des Technol Educ 10:308–319

Lamb JM, Kallal MJ (1992) A conceptual framework for apparel design. Cloth Text Res J 10:42–47

Martin B, Hanington B (2012) Universal methods of design. Rockport, Beverly

McCracken G (1988) Culture and consumption: new approaches to the symbolic character of consumer goods and activities. Indiana University Press, Bloomington

Miller D (2005) Introduction. In: Miller D (ed) Materiality. Duke University Press, Durham

Norman DA (2005) Emotional design: why we love (or hate) everyday things. Basic Books, New York

Partington A (2014) Class, clothes, and co-creativity. Cloth Cult 1:7–21

Ryan M (1966) Clothing: a study in human behavior. Holt, Rinehart & Winston, New York
Spence J (2001) Flying on one wing. In: Guy A, Green E, Banim M (eds) Through the wardrobe: women's relationships with their clothes. Berg, New York
Stone GP (1962) Appearance and the self. In: Rose AM (ed) Human behavior and social process. Houghton-Mifflin, Boston
Story MF (2001) Principles of universal design. In: Preiser WFE, Ostroff E (eds) Universal design handbook. McGraw-Hill, New York
Tseëlon E (1995) The masque of femininity: the presentation of woman in everyday life. Sage, London
Tullio-Pow S, Schaefer K, Nyhof-Young J (2011a) Inclusive post-mastectomy sleepwear: toward sweet dreams for all. In: Paper presented at the international textile and apparel association conference, Philadelphia, PA, US, November
Tullio-Pow S, Schaefer K, Zhu R, Kolenchenko O, Nyhof-Young J (2011b) Sweet dreams: needs assessment and prototype design of post-mastectomy sleepwear. In: Proceedings of Include 2011, Royal College of Art, London, UK, 18–20 April 2011
Twigg J (2013) Fashion and age: dress, the body and later life. Bloomsbury, London
Winkler WA (1977) Choosing the prosthesis and clothing. Am J Nurs 77:1433–1436
Woodward S (2007) Why women wear what they wear. Bloomsbury, London

'Innova' Digital Application and Database for Designers to Innovate for Carers

M. Strickfaden(✉), C. Fiorentino, M. Martin, J. Eales, and J. Fast

Department of Human Ecology, University of Alberta, Edmonton, AB, Canada
megan.strickfaden@ualberta.ca

Abstract. This paper reports on the interdisciplinary design, development, and implementation of a digital application and database called '*Innova*' that serves as a platform to collect and analyse assistive technologies (AT) currently available for family/friend carers and consequently also care recipients. AT products/systems/services that support carers (directly or indirectly) in their everyday lives have the potential to serve as precedents to inform innovators to create new AT products/systems/services to better meet the needs of carers. These precedents become 'materialised design knowledge' that is a significant kit of information that acts as sources of inspiration for designers. The aim of *Innova* is to compile and examine information about AT precedents as a precedent-based design (PBD) tool for designers to improve and/or create new AT products/systems/services that better suit carers' needs. *Innova* is a digital environment that includes an application and database that can be used on Android smartphones and tablets. The digital application and database have a user-centered survey, a user-interface, and feedback features to collect information about AT precedents.

1 Introduction

The design, development and implementation of *Innova* was initiated by bringing together interdisciplinary knowledge about carers, caring and designing. Decades of research highlight the burden of care (e.g., Keating et al. 2014; Keating and Eales 2017), the lack of products available that directly support caring for older adults or patients with acute conditions, and support an in-depth examination of the product-types that are currently available on the market for patients and carers. The end-user of *Innova*—carers who would be inputting AT products into the digital application/database and the designers who would be using the AT products in the database as sources of inspiration—were consulted throughout the process. However, this evidence-based design approach and consultations are not the focus of this paper. Here the focus is on the dynamic process of development that happens when a team of people from diverse disciplines is brought together in the naming, visual identity, visual design guidelines of *Innova*; and the programming of *Innova*.

The design and development of *Innova* demanded an interdisciplinary effort that brought together a team of experts, scholars and students from diverse backgrounds.

P. Langdon et al. (Eds.): CWUAAT 2020, *Designing for Inclusion*, pp. 35–46, 2020.
https://doi.org/10.1007/978-3-030-43865-4_4

These were composed of an AGE-WELL[1] pool of experts and scholars (project leads, collaborators, supervisors) as well as trainees, known as highly qualified personnel (HQPs), from the areas of human ecology, gerontology, aging studies, material culture, and visual communication design. Additionally, a team of students in the areas of computing science and human ecology were involved in developing the first version of *Innova*.

Innova is a precedent-based design (PBD) research tool in the form of digital application and database that can be used on Android smartphones and tablets. As a PBD tool, *Innova* aids designers with the research process by supporting innovation towards new products/systems/services by identifying what already exists and prevents designers from 're-inventing the wheel'. As such, the guiding question for the work presented here is: *What innovative technological solutions already exist in the market or are being developed for the industry to address caregivers' needs?*

Motivation for developing *Innova* was that there is little information available about what assistive technologies (AT) products/systems/services are currently available for carers in Canada (and globally) and our team had the assumption that there were actually few innovations specifically geared towards carers as the target user-group. Ongoing scans of AT products/systems/services revealed numerous items available for care recipients, medical professionals including occupational and physiotherapists, and doctors, and fewer AT products/systems/services for carers. Innova's content involves building up a library of existing AT through having different kinds of AT users and producers input specific examples with accompanying information about these products/systems/services.

The information about AT products/systems/services includes quantitative (e.g., demographics, technical specifications, dimensions, price) and qualitative (e.g., materials, performance, user comments, photographs of the product) details. The information is further stored in a database accessed through a website (Fig. 1).

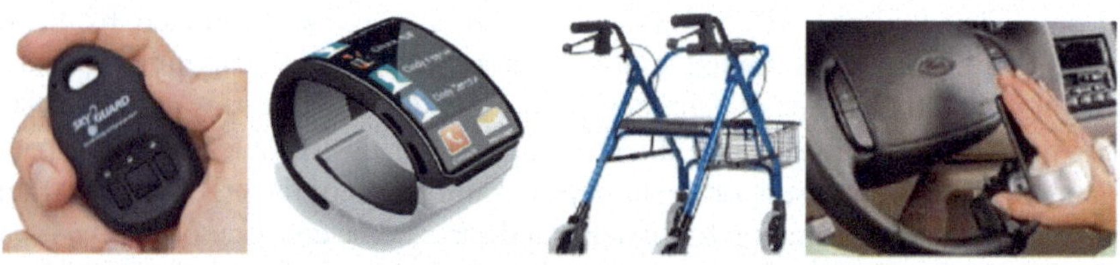

Fig. 1. Examples of *Innova's* content of AT devices

Innova, therefore, acts as a set of "inspirational sources" (e.g., Eckert and Stacey 2000; Strickfaden et al. 2015) to encourage precedent based design (PBD) that is defined as "the process of the selection of relevant concepts from prior designs in order to apply ideas and conceptual solutions to current design situations" (Oxman and Oxman 1993,

[1] AGE-WELL NCE (Aging Gracefully across Environments using Technology to Support Wellness, Engagement and Long Life NCE Inc.) is Canada's technology and aging network, dedicated to the creation of technologies and services that benefit older adults and carers. Launched in 2015 through the federally-funded.

p. 55). PBD originated from case-based reasoning (CBR), a computing method characterised as a problem-solving approach, useful for retrieving and indexing information for PBD (Oxman 1996). Various PBD databases have been developed including, for example, case-based design tools for architectural designers (Heylighen and Neuckermans 2001). In short, PBD is a library of products/systems/services that are a kind of 'materialised design knowledge' that is a significant kit of information that acts as sources of inspiration for designers[2]. Identifying and observing precedents as part of design research is known to prevent ill-formulated processes that avoid redundancy in design which in turn benefits clients and end-users by providing more refined and relevant products/systems/services.

This paper identifies the rationale for focusing on designers and carers as our target user groups, the need to design more products/systems/services for carers, and a definition of AT products/services. This is followed with a detailed and rich description of the two parts of *Innova* as a designed product. We continue with reports on the interdisciplinary design and development of a digital application (front end) and database (back end) are created. This interdisciplinary development includes defining the three groups who worked on *Innova*, and the naming, visual identity, visual design guidelines and programming of *Innova*.

2 Background

Worldwide, family and friends provide the vast majority of care to people with chronic health conditions, disabilities or aging-related needs. These carers represent a significant segment of the population: 43.5 million Americans (National Alliance for Caregiving and AARP 2015), 8.1 million Canadians (Sinha 2012), 6.5 million people in the UK (Carers UK 2015) and 2.7 million Australians (Carers Australia 2015). Carers have unique needs; they often experience health, social and economic consequences as a result of their care taking roles (Keating et al. 2014; Keating and Eales 2017). Assistive Technologies (AT) are assumed to lighten the burden of carers (Pollack 2005; Bharucha et al. 2009; Topo 2009), yet Sheets et al. (2014) argues for "comprehensive assessment and person-centered approaches to meet caregiver needs". Encompassing this trend, there is an increasing demand for AT that supports carers and care recipients and a need to assess what innovative technological solutions currently exist.

For the purpose of this paper and to design and develop *Innova,* AT are defined as any product (e.g., tool, piece of equipment), system, and/or service that achieves one or more of the following for family/friend carers:

1. Reduces physical and/or psychological burden;
2. Allows for choice in the activities caregivers carry out in their daily lives;
3. Supports, maintains and/or improves, autonomy privacy, dignity, participation, and engagement in daily, social, and entertainment activities, and/or functional capabilities;
4. Increases safety and/or health monitoring;
5. Provides information that assists all of the above.

[2] Designers refer to product developers and engineers, industrial designers, graphic designers, and any other innovators who could benefit from PBD.

Communicating caregiver needs to AT designers is a crucial step to developing effective technological solutions. An approach that serves to aid in developing AT begins with the need to provide access to information about technologies known to be useful to carers in comprehensive and reliable ways. This is addressed through *Innova* by assessing existing technological solutions on the market through PBD.

3 'Innova' Digital Application and Database

For the implementation of a PBD digital application and database it was necessary to design a tool capable of storing rich and detailed information that is made accessible to designers of current and future AT products/systems/services. The *Innova* digital application and database focuses on:

1. Bringing a design perspective to the information collected;
2. Highlighting currently available AT products, systems and services;
3. Critically analysing available AT products, systems and services;
4. Discovering gaps, including poorly-designed and unavailable AT products, systems and services;
5. Making information about AT products, systems and services accessible to the communities of carers, designers, and producers.

3.1 How Does Innova Work?

Innova is a digital application and database that is currently a closed system. The system has two interfaces: through an application that is designed for Android smartphones and tablets (front-end) and a database accessed through any digital source (back-end). These two interfaces operate at two ends of the system: first by collecting information through a type of survey (the application/front-end) and second by processing and administrating the collected information (the database/back-end) (see Fig. 2).

The front-end and back-end interfaces respond to two different targeted users. The front-end is geared towards carers who use AT products/systems/services, AT producers, AT designers and other random AT users (e.g., researchers, technologists, students). Each of these user groups need to be able to provide information about one or more specific AT product/system/service by completing the survey on the application. The back-end is geared towards administrators and researchers involved in the development of *Innova,* but may also be of interest to other researchers, designers, and/or producers. A third component of this closed system will be a future development in the form of a website that will contain results and relevant details of the collected AT cases.

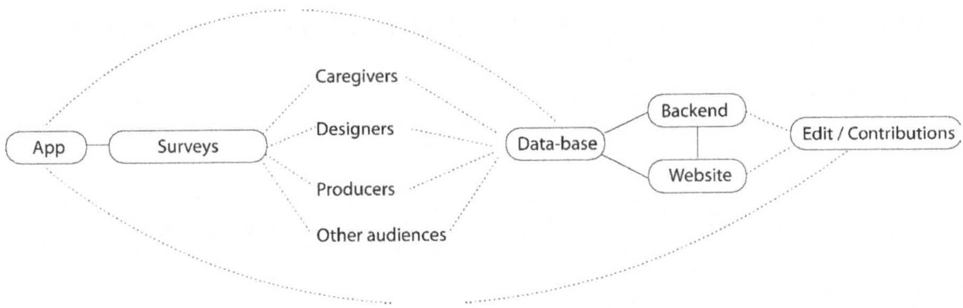

Fig. 2. *Innova's* closed system with front-end and back-end interfaces

The sequence that *Innova's* closed system is as follows:

1. A user is invited to participate or find the application available to install on a handset device (smart phone or tablet),
2. The user opens the application and fills a form with basic information that is stored in the database. This information helps to determine what kind of user is providing information (carer, designer, producer, other). The inquiries are complemented with definitions of various kinds of equipment, products, systems and services.
3. Once basic information is provided, the user is asked to provide details of a single AT product, system or service. Questions about these AT examples or cases are formulated in the form of multiple-choice questions. A user can also provide additional comments, descriptions and critiques. The application guides the user over these steps sequentially, however the user can move back and forth in the process by changing responses, jumping ahead, and skipping questions.
4. Along with conventional details (e.g., weblinks) about AT products/systems/services the user can add their own photograph or a sketch. Photographs can be copy-pasted from an existing source (photo album, website, etc.) or can be taken through the device's camera. For sketching, an embedded drawing tool with options on line values and colours is included.
5. When the user completes all the information, and presses the "submit" button, the data is sent to the database. Administrators and researchers can access the uploaded information in real time through the back-end.
6. The database interface is accessed as a digital desktop environment or can be exported as standard tables to be opened in most conventional spread-sheet software. The database also creates dynamic distribution and impact charts, and other visualisations to support the analysis of the information obtained.
7. The information obtained through the database supports identifying opportunities, limitations and gaps in current AT products/systems/services.

3.2 Front-End Target User Group

Understanding the intended target user group of *Innova* provided key elements to shape its interface design. The four target users are defined as family/friend carers, designers, producers and others. 'Family/friend carers' are those individuals who provide unpaid help or care to a family member or friend with a long-term health condition, physical or mental disability or aging-related needs because of a personal relationship with that person. 'Designers' are professional practitioners who are able to create and/or analyse artifacts. Artefacts are two- and three-dimensional things such as prototypes, final products or services, and end-user documentation. 'Producers' are experts in the industry who work collaboratively with managers, designers, and engineering teams in the process of manufacturing or production of objects. The 'others' category is for people who are care receivers, paid caregivers, healthcare practitioners or providers, researchers or those who are not solely a family caregiver, a designer or producer. That is, the user may have multiple roles, such as family/friend carer and designer.

4 Interdisciplinary Development of 'Innova'

The interdisciplinary team of experts, scholars and students involved in creating *Innova* can be synthesised in three groups with different dynamics:

1. Group 1 included the AGEWELL experts, scholars and HQPs with expertise in aging, caregiving and AT for older adults, and the design team with expertise in design processes, inspiration and influence, innovation, PBD, CBR, product engineering and graphic design. This group focused on the goal of developing the content and details of *Innova*.
2. Group 2 included the design (the same design team as in group 1) and the student application and database developers guided by a seasoned computer scientist. These experts, scholars, HQPs and students were in charge of programming the application and database.
3. Group 3 included all the team members in groups 1 and 2 in testing the final *Innova* prototype.

Group dynamics demanded rich dialoguing across disciplines and the development of a common language to achieve the objectives of *Innova* that went through a number of iterations. The common language was materialised in a tangible result (the application and database created) that provided the foundations for further research.

4.1 Design and Development Process

The design process of *Innova* began with researching and developing content. Group 1 worked together to establish some essential basics in order to further the project. Therefore, the overall research goals for Innova were determined first to create a focus for the project. These included:

1. Identifying assistive technologies (AT) that are currently available to family/friend carers.
2. Collecting carers' evaluations and critical reviews of existing AT products/systems/services including how those AT products/systems/services are defined. This goal also involves identifying carers needs, wants, desires and expectations.

3. Making descriptive, evaluative and critical information about AT products/systems /services publically available.
4. Give access to designers and producers to the precedents collected in *Innova*, and inform them about the unmet AT needs of carers, so that cutting edge AT can be designed to enhance carers well-being.

The interdisciplinary design and development process of creating *Innova* included a dynamic and unique process. Group 1, 2 and 3 were involved in the design and development process in order to achieve the above four goals. Ten core steps are summarised:

(1) Develop the data collection survey;
(2) Design a visual identity for *Innova*;
(3) Implement the visual identity to the interface design;
(4) Design the interfaces for the application and database;
(5) Participate in the development of the application, database and interface programming;
(6) Follow-up with the data entry process and preliminary analysis to test early versions of *Innova*;
(7) Create visualisations for the information collected that can display these to designers and producers;
(8) Conduct target user group testing;
(9) Refine the design details of the application and database;
(10) Participate in new collaborative AT product/system/service design projects.

4.2 Naming, Visual Identity and Visual Design Guidelines

The design, development, and implementation of *Innova* naturally required the development of a name, a visual identity and design guidelines to ensure the interfaces of the application and database were well-received by the user groups. A visual communication approach was coordinated with the content design and development of *Innova*. Naming *Innova* and creating a visual identity involved research (what names were already used? What were the connotations of various names? etc.). A long list of names was logged. Second to naming *Innova* was developing a language of typography and colour. Five main variations of typography and colour were considered, and more than twenty logo versions were developed. The chosen name and logo was *Innova* (Fig. 3). The name *Innova* stands for 'innovation' and 'assistance'.

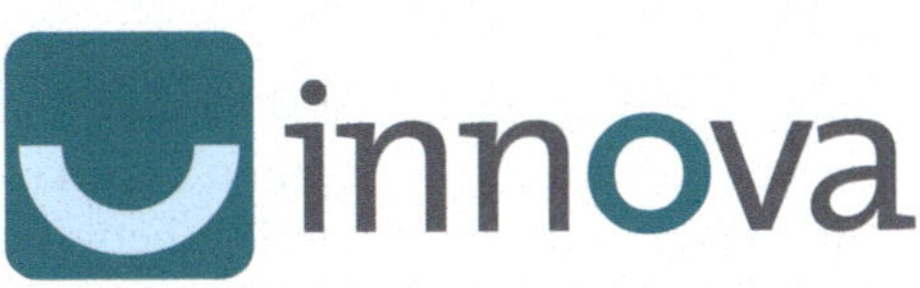

Fig. 3. Logo design by Carlos Fiorentino

The visual elements developed for *Innova* are a colour palette based on teal and blue. The logo development is based mainly on a play with typography (Fig. 4).

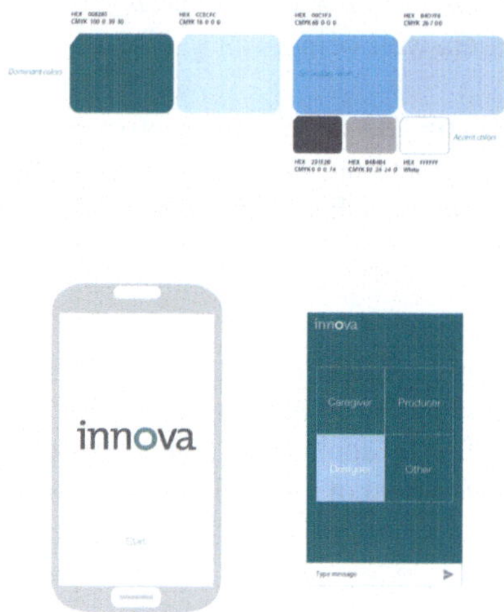

Fig. 4. Details of colour and typology designed by Carlos Fiorentino

Innova's logo emphasises the 'o' and includes a curved 'smile that adds a playful and friendly character to the visual identity. The family of typefaces used for the logo is *Thesis Mix*, while *Helvetica* (or alternatively *Arial* and *Roboto*) are options for system fonts in labels and general text. The balance between graphic elements conveys the idea of a friendly-intuitive aesthetic that also feels like a rigorous research tool.

Prior to working with group 2 on the programming of the application and database for *Innova*, visual design guidelines were created. These were created in order to collaboratively guide group 2 and to ensure a high quality finished product. The visual design guidelines comprised of the main graphic elements, basic screen typologies, and basic rules for implementation. The visual design guidelines initially focused on the interfaces related to the application for Android smartphones and tablets. The screen typologies show how the visual identity for *Innova* was developed following the general rules of these guidelines. Group 2 worked closely together in the development stages that were iterative and involved numerous meetings and extensive dialoguing to implement the visual identity.

4.3 Programming

Along with creating a naming and developing visual identity and visual design guidelines, the programming of *Innova* continued with group 2 working together. The front-end application for Android devices works as the interface between the information input of the target user groups and the back-end database that contains information analyses functions for designers, producers and administration. These two main components of *Innova* were the focus of programming and development. The programming team made decisions and coded to ensure a product that suited the goals and content defined by group 1. This programming process required regular meetings between the developers and designers, regular rounds of sketching and mock-up versions of the tool, running prototypes, and final checkups, testing and follow-up stages, until they obtained a final version of the application and database. The two main goals for the team of developers were:

1. Create a dynamic and flexible questionnaire application to gather information about AT (front-end).
2. Post all the information to a database where it would be overseen by administration and statistics could be collected (back-end).

Front-End Application: The team of developers had to consider three key metrics for the Android application front-end: the capacity to support Android 4.0 ICS to 6.0 Marshmallow operating system; the opportunity to use the vast coverage of Android devices (97.3%); and the need of a responsive design for Android smartphones and tablets.

The resulting application interface is based on 'Google Material Design Lite Guidelines'. The tool required a dynamic flow that considers:

(a) Future question sequences depending on previous answers;
(b) Researcher capability to skip and redirect results.

To address the complexity of the interface system, three main technologies were used to develop the application:

(1) JSON (JavaScript Object Notation) a lightweight technology for data exchange;
(2) Question storage, a capacity of the system to saving and simplifying communication with the server;
(3) Gson (Persistence) a Java library that converts data from JSON representation.

Back-End Database: The backend database (Fig. 5) consists of two main components: the database where the data is stored in a server; and the interface to access, modify and administrate that data. Both components are essential for the functionality of the database.

In other words, the database cannot be used without a back-end interface that provides access to the data stored, and a back-end interface has no purpose if there is no database to access. The back-end database provides a graphical interface with general statistics that is easy read by designers and producers. The back-end database developers identified three key challenges that were addressed:

1. User authentication and session management versatility: For this challenge developers created an administrative login function to access the back-end interface.

2. Search through questionnaire submissions: The developers created a back-end interface, basically functioning as a simple website structure, which allows administrators and researchers to read in detail the submitted responses to the app questionnaire. The interface is also capable of showing generated statistics from the data collected from questionnaires (as shown in Fig. 3).
3. Questionnaire versioning: the different targeted audiences considered for *Innova* required different versions of the questionnaire, in which the order and content of the questions can be easily changed, tracked and analysed. Updates to the questions were also frequently required. Developers created a method that facilitates this process in the backend.

The database development was based on the following coding technologies:

1. MEAN Stack
2. Node.js (HTTP Server)
3. Express.js (Web App Framework)
4. HTML5, JS, CSS3 (Front-end, standard)
5. Angular.js (MVC Framework)
6. MongoDB (Database)

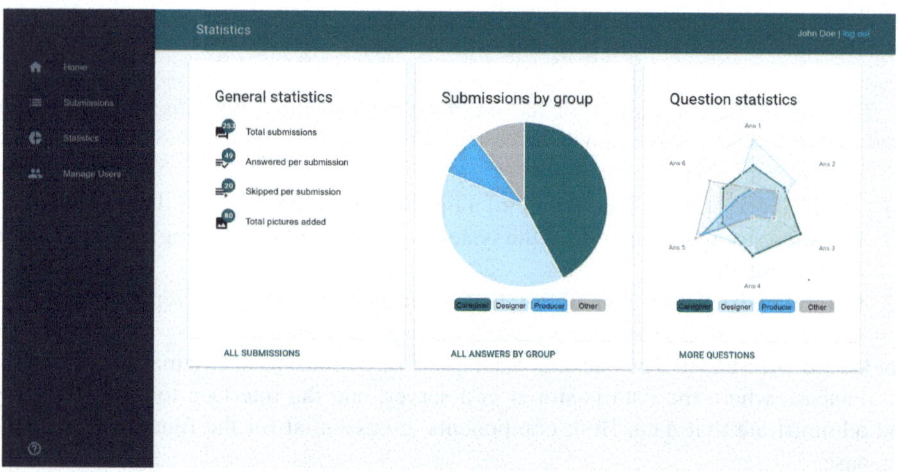

Fig. 5. Screenshot of the back-end database and administration homepage

5 Conclusion

Our design, development, and implementation of *Innova's* digital application and database has been informed by similar projects that engage in interaction design (e.g., Banga and Weinhold 2014), multi-device experiences (e.g., Levin 2014), and user-centred design practices (Jordan 2001; Iny 2018). Even so, this paper has emphasised interdisciplinarity and complexity as part of the process by highlighting the myriad of considerations, research, decisions, and aspects of collaborative practice required to reach a final product. We acknowledge that building an application and database to collect AT products/systems/services to be used for PBD can be a long-term quest; however, the use of this resource can also be progressive and requires imagining the future use of the product and extensive user testing. We also acknowledge that *Innova* is a dynamic product that grows and enriches in quality when consulted and used by carers, designers, AT producers and other professionals. Furthermore, ongoing user testing is also a significant part of the design, development and implementation of *Innova*.

As a product that has the potential to help designers generate innovative products/systems/services, *Innova* is expected to grow as a system and expand its capabilities and gain a broader audience by adding new components. Although the application is currently available on Android, we believe it should be available for iOS (Apple devices) as well as in website form to be accessed from any browser. This would provide greater access resulting in a wider range and bigger number of cases for designers and producers to peruse. The website would also contain more detailed information about the AT products/systems/services, the outcomes, and the research community involved in AT for older adults.

Innova—as a system that includes an application, database, website—is in the process of being commercialised. As it stands, *Innova*'s database offers features for designers and researchers, such as statistics and other ways to visualise information, but we hope this can be expanded in the future. In the process of commercialisation we are hopeful that *Innova* will be linked to other databases so it can be populated with a larger number of AT products/systems/services including ones that are available on the market and ones that are speculative.

Acknowledgements. The authors gratefully acknowledge the financial contributions of AGE-WELL NCE Ltd., Canada's technology and aging network, through the core research project WP2.4 Assistive Technology that Cares for the Caregiver.

References

Banga C, Weinhold J (2014) Essential mobile interaction design: perfecting interface design in mobile apps. Addison-Wesley (Pearson Education), Boston

Bharucha AJ, Anand V, Forlizzi J, Dew MA et al (2009) Intelligent assistive technology applications to dementia care: current capabilities, limitations, and future challenges. Am J Geriatr Psychiatry 17(2):88–104

Carers Australia (2015). www.carersaustralia.com.au/about-carers/statistics/. Accessed 18 Dec 2019

Carers UK (2015). www.carersuk.org/news-and-campaigns/press-releases/facts-and-figures. Accessed 2 Aug 2017

Eckert C, Stacey M (2000) Sources of inspiration: a language of design. Des Stud 21:523–538

Heylighen A, Neuckermans H (2001) A case base of case-based design tools for architecture. Comput Aided Des 33(14):1111–1122

Iny C (2018) The best UX tools for user research and user testing, 2019 Edition. UsabilityGeek. 2011–19. usabilitygeek.com/best-ux-tools-user-research-user-testing-2018/. Accessed 16 Dec 2019

Jordan P (2001) An introduction to usability. Taylor & Francis Inc., Philadelphia
Keating N, Eales J (2017) Social consequences of family care: a scoping review. Int J Care Caring 1(2):153–173
Keating NC, Fast JE, Lero DS, Lucas SJ, Eales J (2014) A taxonomy of the economic costs of family care to adults. J Econ Ageing 3:11–20
Levin M (2014) Designing multi-device experiences: an ecosystem approach to user experiences across devices. O'Reilly Media, Inc., Sebastopol
National Alliance for Caregiving and AARP (2015). www.caregiving.org/wp-content/uploads/2015/05/2015_CaregivingintheUS_Final-Report-June-4_WEB.pdf. Accessed 2 Aug 2017
Oxman R, Oxman R (1993) Precedents: memory structure in design case libraries. In: Flemming U, Van Wyk S (eds) CAAD futures 1993. Elsevier Science Publishers, Amsterdam
Oxman R (1996) Case-based design support: supporting architectural composition through precedent libraries. J Archit Plan Res 13(3):242–255
Pollack M (2005) Intelligent technology for an aging population: the use of AI to assist elders with cognitive impairment. AI Mag 26(2):9
Sheets D, Black K, Kaye L (2014) Who cares for caregivers? Evidence-based approaches to family support. J Gerontol Soc Work 57(6–7):525–530
Sinha M (2012) Analytical paper. Spotlight on Canadians: Results from the general social survey. Portrait of caregivers, 2012. Statistics Canada, Ottawa, Canada. www.statcan.gc.ca/pub/89-652-x/89-652-x2013001-eng.pdf. Accessed 2 Aug 2017
Strickfaden M, Stafiniak L, Terzin T (2015) Inspired and inspiring designers: understanding creativity through influence and inspiration. Cloth Text Res J 33(3):213–228
Topo P (2009) Technology studies to meet the needs of people with dementia and their caregivers: a literature review. J Appl Gerontol 28(1):5–37

The Co-creation Process of a Platform for Healthcare Engineering Design and Innovation (HEDI)

L. Liu[1], Y. Jiang[1(✉)], H. Dong[2], T. C. Lee[1], and Q. Y. Liu[1]

[1] College of Design and Innovation, Tongji University, Shanghai, China
liulong@tongji.edu.cn, tju_joey@163.com, taklee@live.com, 634448077@qq.com

[2] School of Design and Creative Arts, Loughborough University, Loughborough, UK
H.Dong@lboro.ac.uk

Abstract. The HEDI platform stands for the Healthcare Engineering Design and Innovation; it is a proposed platform aimd to promote co-creation of medical products with cooperation of different stakeholders with specialised expertise.

Co-creation activities can be conducted either offline or online. In this study, The offline co-creation mechanisms were tested through three projects to gain insights into what worked and what did not work. Online co-creation platforms such as Quirky, Kaizao were analysed to summerise their attributes.

Based on the investigation of offline co-creation methanisms and online co-creation platforms, insights were drawn for the development of the co-creation platform of HEDI. The Value-Methodology-Execution (VME) Pyramid was used to illustrate the structure and significance of co-creation for healthcare engineering design and innovation.

1 Introduction

Modern medical services are increasingly dependent on a variety of medical products and systems. At the same time, in the process of diagnosis and treatment, there is an increasing need for patient-centred design of product and service, which provides designers many opportunities as well as challenges when facing this highly specialised industry sector.

In China, with high economy development and the rapid increase in demands for high-quality modern healthcare service, there is a need for safer and more effective medical products. The relevant government departments, medical industries, and medical-related design organisations are all motivated to explore better means for medical product design and development. As the traditional Chinese medical product manufacturers have, for a long time, adopted a technology-driven approach for medical product design, the requirements of end users (as patients or healthcare providers) are often poorly considered in the process (Weinger et al. 2010). User-centred design of medical products is not the norm. Instead, the most common design process is dominated by engineers and lacks collaboration between different stakeholders or disciplines, which significantly reduces the effectiveness and efficiency of the design process because many specific needs of the end users are not well investigated or incorporated into design.

P. Langdon et al. (Eds.): CWUAAT 2020, *Designing for Inclusion*, pp. 47–55, 2020.
https://doi.org/10.1007/978-3-030-43865-4_5

Medical product design is a special design sector which needs specialised expertise, multi-disciplinary cooperation, iterative design and evaluation with participation of end users. It has a very high threshold for most of the designers to enter as they are not capable of getting sufficient professional experiences within a short period of time (Ham et al. 2003). Because of the difference in mental model of designers, healthcare providers, and patients, a co-creation approach should be adopted as a better solution to medical product design (Sanders and Stappers 2008).

Based on the understanding of the current problem, we propose to establish an online co-creation platform to promote the interaction of different stakeholders of medial product design. This platform of Healthcare Engineering Design and Innovation (HEDI) focuses on the healthcare sector with co-creation methods and tools to assist the interaction between different stakeholders. This paper presents our studies on identifying appropriate co-creation principles to define and design the HEDI platform. VME Pyramid is developed to illustrate the structure and significance of co-creation for healthcare engineering design and innovation.

2 Offline Co-creation Practice

Co-creation activities can be conducted either offline or online. We firstly tested offline co-creation mechanisms through practical projects to gain insights into what worked and what did not work.

2.1 Co-creation with Doctors in the Medical Lab

The first project was conducted in November 2018 as a survey in the Basic Clinical Medical Lab at Tongji University, Shanghai, China. The aim of this study was to understand the healthcare practice from the designers' point of view, and to identify co-creation opportunities of designers with doctors and medical students.

Our observation in the medical lab revealed that the healthcare professionals did not obey the intended use mode of some devices in practice. Figure 1 shows an example. After a medical experiment, a variety of equipment used frequently was randomly inserted in a foam container on the table (as shown on the right image) instead of being placed as designed (as shown on the left image). The medical students in the Lab had their own preferred way of laying out the instruments, not following certain Medical Lab Regulations (e.g., Yetisen et al. 2014) which require that different items to be categorised and put in different containers. This had posed risks in use, providing an interesting design opportunity for co-creation for improvement.

2.2 Co-creation with Local Residents for NICE 2035

The second project was the co-creation of an art mural in a community (shown in Fig. 2). More than 100 local residents ranging from 5-year-olds to 80-year-olds were involved in creating a 30-m long mural with black and white paint. This allowed the participants to freely express their imagination and their voice of the future community. The co-creation was organised by designers with the combination of offline and online mechanisms.

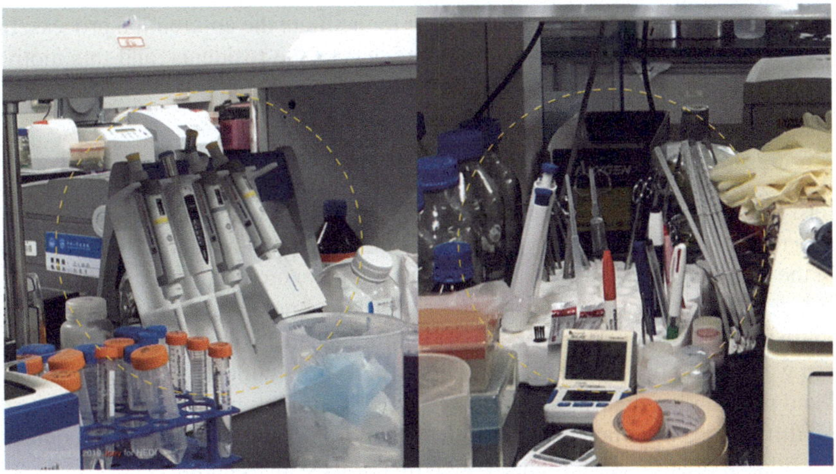

Fig. 1. Toolbox vs. the foam container in the basic medical lab

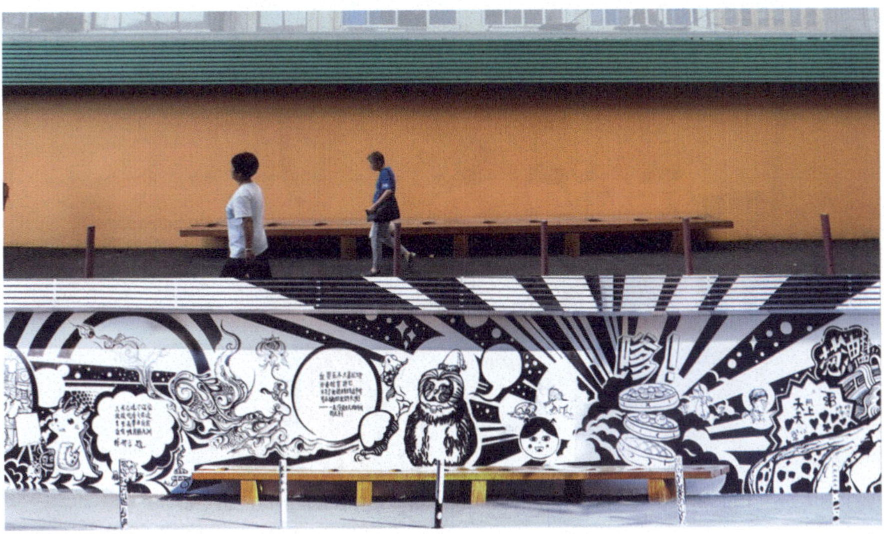

Fig. 2. Co-creation of an art mural at a community with designers and ordinary people

The online promotion attracted more than fifty thousand readings and some ideas were developed and integrated into the mural design. With an initial pattern provided to trigger imagination, the mural was gradually finished with the participation of both residents and designers on site, in three days.

From this co-creation project we understood the strength of using the online platform for idea collection: it was cost-effective, and had little time or space limit. The online platform provided the dynamic interaction of designers with ordinary people.

The visualisation support was a key factor to facilitate the co-creation process. In the mural project, designers helped visualise the ideas of the residents, and this motivated the participation of ordinary people in the co-creation process.

2.3 Co-creation with Children in the Shanghai Children's Medical Centre

The third study was conducted in the Shanghai Children's Medical Centre with in-patient children, to let them create Disney facilities as their dream game and at the same time to relieve the children's nervousness. Gamification tools were used to help the interaction between designers and children. The co-creation was implemented in the play room of this centre with two groups of participants (5 children and 2 volunteers in each group, the children were accompanied by their parents) (Fig. 3). As children were quite diverse in mood and personality, their participation effect was difficult to predict. The researchers found it difficult to communicate well with the children to achieve co-creation outcomes, but the children themselves felt happy with this process in general.

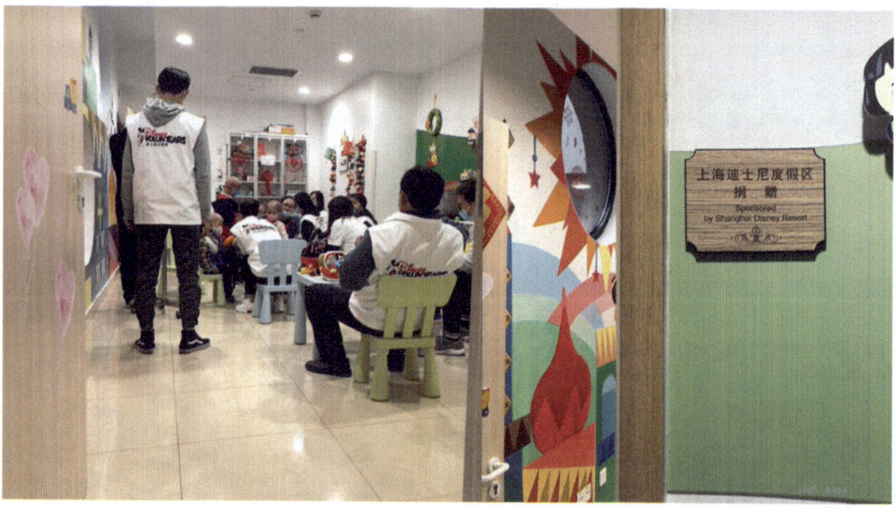
上海迪士尼度假区
捐 赠
Sponsored
by Shanghai Disney Resort

Fig. 3. Co-creation in the Shanghai Children's Medical Centre

The study has shown the challenge of co-creation with young patients who are experiencing subnormal status, physiologically or psychologically. Their motivation, readiness for communication, participation duration, and acceptance of tools, are quite different to other co-creation situations. The effectiveness of offline participation of patients should be further studied.

2.4 Insights from Offline Co-creation Projects

The offline co-creation projects provide us valuable insights into why and how to establish an online platform to support medical product design more effectively. Important insights for HEDI can be summarised below:

- Providing an online platform can help reduce time for offline co-creation. The online platform may have multiple functions such as promotion, motivating participation, inspiring idea, and facilitating interaction.
- An effective online platform to support offline co-creation should have good dynamic features to enhance timely and simultaneous interactions of different parties.
- Many existing regulations in the medical product design sector are unfamiliar to designers, and they are not easy to be discovered by the interaction with healthcare professionals. Better references should be integrated into an on-line platform to inform designers.
- Safe use and risk issues should be well considered with measures in the co-creation process to ensure these issues are not overseen.
- There should be a mechanism to evaluate initial ideas in an effective way.
- Visualisation of initial ideas should be supported to facilitate communication between different parties.
- Typical frameworks of concepts and designs should be formulated to provide a basis for further development with efficiency. The online platform should have embedded learning mechanisms to promote design development.
- The engagement of patients in the co-creation process is critical but difficult. The value of the participation of the patients should be evaluated to ensure their needs are accommodated and reflected in the design process.

3 Online Co-creation Research

Based on the new possible combination of "digitalisation" and "emotionalisation", and with the initial development of Computer Supported Cooperative Work (CSCW), user participation has gradually expanded from offline to online (Yu 2017). Many online co-creation platforms exist and we reviewed some of them.

3.1 Existing Online Co-creation Platforms

Many factors can affect the attributes of an online co-creation platform. If using "Openness" and "Ownership" as the two main factors, with consideration of the secondary factors such as the amount of people involved, competition degree, customer competence, dialogue frequency, project duration, etc., online co-creation platforms can be divided into four types as follows: Crow of people, Community of kindred spirits, Club of experts, and Coalition of parties (Cottam and Leadbeater n.d.; Innolytics n.d.; Manu Vollens n.d.) (Fig. 4).

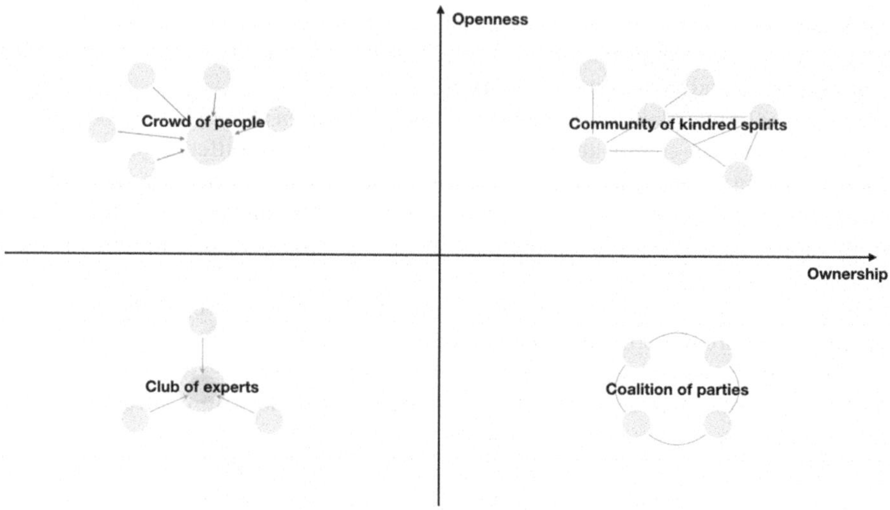

Fig. 4. Category of online co-creation platforms

3.2 Positioning of HEDI

To better assess the potential trends of online co-creation platforms, we conducted a review of 13 existing online co-creation platforms, including Quirky, Brineet, and Kaizao. Table 1 summarises their features, with the researchers' rating of '0–5' of their attributes (0 means none, 1 means low and 5 means high). We re-categorised them according to the framework mentioned above (shown in Fig. 5). Using this framework to indicate the positioning of HEDI, we may place HEDI in the first quadrant closer to the right end of the Ownership-axis, which means that it has a medium degree of openness with a high degree of ownership by both the initiators and contributors in the co-creation projects.

Table 1. Features of co-creation platforms

Website	Category	No. of people involved	Customer competence	Return for participants	Competition degree
Blue Sky Lab	Club of experts	3	4	2	1
Braineet	Crowd of people	5	5	5	4
CITYNET	Coalition of parties	4	4	4	1
Flemish Living Lab Platform	Club of experts	2	1	3	0
harKopen	Community of kindred spirits	5	4	2	0
Innocentive	Crowd of people	3	5	3	4

(continued)

Table 1. (*continued*)

Website	Category	No. of people involved	Customer competence	Return for participants	Competition degree
Jovoto	Community of kindred spirits	4	4	5	3
Kaizao	Community of kindred spirits	4	3	4	1
Open IDEO	Crowd of people	4	1	2	3
Quirky	Crowd of people	5	4	5	4
Redesignme	Crowd of people	4	3	4	5
SloCat	Coalition of parties	4	4	4	1
Ushahidi	Community of kindred spirits	5	1	2	0

Note that, the factor "number of people involved" and "Customer Competence" are linked with "Openness"; And the factor "Return for Participants" and "Competition Degree" are linked with "Ownership".

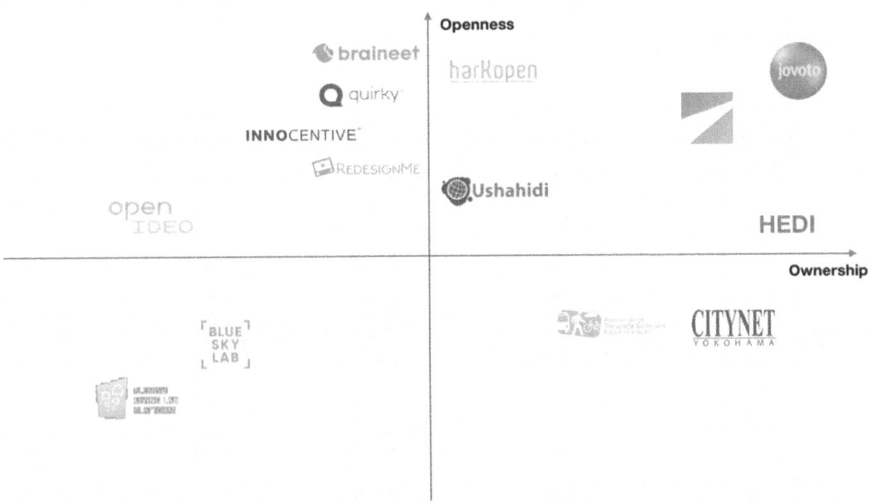

Fig. 5. Positioning of existing co-creation platforms and HEDI

4 Value-Methodology-Execution Pyramid

Based on the investigation of three offline co-creation projects and the review of online co-creation platforms, with consideration of the objective of the HEDI platform, we defined fundamental features of HEDI. With the help of the VME Pyramid, these features could be illustrated to show the structure of the HEDI platform (Fig. 6). Based on this VME Pyramid, it is possible to plan further studies for the HEDI platform to coordinate different stakeholders (healthcare professionals, patients, designers, enigineers, etc.) to co-create user-centric medical products and services.

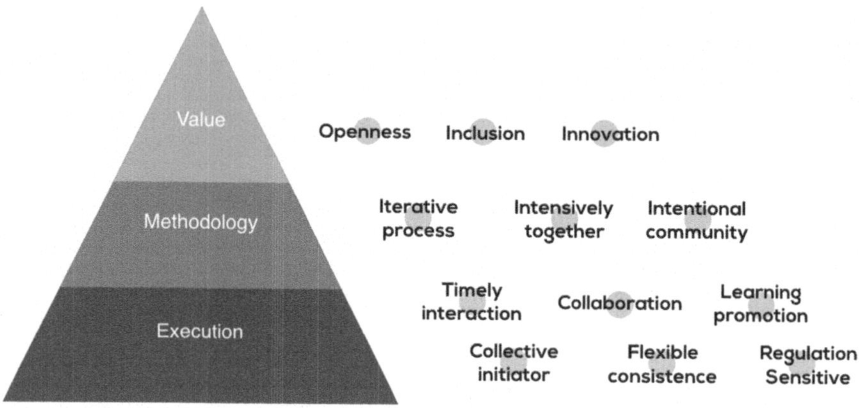

Fig. 6. The VME Pyramid of HEDI

5 Conclusion and Future Work

Design in the healthcare sector has its unique charecteristic. As most designers are not familiar with the highly specialised requirements, the collaboration of different parties with multi-disciplinary backgrounds is essential to ensure the effectiveness of medical product design. Co-creation approaches are a good solution to mitigate the problem posed by the exclusion of end users (e.g., healthcare providers and patients) from the design process. This paper presents some initial results of the studies to establish the online platform of HEDI for medical product design. The VME Pyramid was developed to illustrate the specification of the platform, which also acted as the guidance for the next steps of study, especially on the following topics:

1. The communication mode of different parties in a real design project. This is the core of the co-creation mechanism specified in HEDI to embody its value. The role and relationship of the designers and the end users in the process should be well studied;
2. The combination of online and offline activities in the co-creation process. This is essential in the implementation of a real co-creation project to plan different activities in a suitable way. A good balance and connection of both should be achieved.
3. The incorporation of regulatory requirements in the co-creation process. This is an unique characteristic of HEDI as in the design process many regulations should be considered.

In the near future, a prototype of HEDI will be developed as the basis for a functional online co-creation platform. The prototype will also realise the mechanism of tracing the contribution of different participants in the co-creation process.

References

Cottam H, Leadbeater C (2004) Health: co-creating services. RED Paper 01. The Design Council, London, UK (2004)

Ham C, Kipping R, McLeod H (2003) Redesigning work processes in healthcare: lessons from the National Health Service. Milbank Q 81(3):415–439

Innolytics (n.d.) Open Innovation Whitepaper. Innolytics

Vollens M (n.d.) How to kickstart your co-creation platform. Board of Innovation

Sanders EBN, Stappers PJ (2008) Co-creation and the new landscapes of design. CoDesign 4(1):5–18

Weinger MB, Wiklund ME, Gardner-Bonneau DJ (2010) Handbook of human factors in medical device design. CRC Press, Boca Raton

Yetisen AK, Martinez-Hurtado JL, da Cruz Vasconcellos F et al (2014) The regulation of mobile medical applications. Lab Chip 14(5):833–840

Measuring Product Demand and Peoples' Capabilities

Patients' Experience of Waiting for Surgery

L. Begley(✉) and H. Dong

School of Design and Creative Arts, Loughborough University, Loughborough, UK
laracatrina31@icloud.com, H.Dong@lboro.ac.uk

Abstract. Waiting times were the most cited reason for dissatisfaction with the UK's National Health Services. Long waits can have a negative impact on a person's health-related quality of life. This study used visual methods and interviews to get insights into patients' experience of waiting for surgery. Five themes were identified through investigating the whole journey leading to an operation: i.e. process, information and communication, autonomy and control, the 'actual experience of waiting', and impact. Data mapping results in four key insights which give direction for future intervention to improve patients' experience of waiting for surgery.

1 Introduction

Waiting times for surgery are a growing concern for publicly funded health services. In July 2018, the total number of patients on waiting lists for surgery on the UK's National Health Service (NHS) reached a 10 year high at 4.3 million patients (Campbell 2018). This has resulted in an increased number of people having to wait more than the target maximum of 18 weeks from referral to treatment. In 2018, waiting times were the most cited reason for dissatisfaction with the NHS, appearing in 52% of survey responses (Robertson et al. 2019).

Long waits can have a negative impact on a person's health-related quality of life (Derrett et al. 1999). Generally, longer wait times are seen as less acceptable, particularly for patients with more severe symptoms such as pain and instability (Carr et al. 2009).

A recent study by the Patient and Client Council (2018) examining the experiences of people waiting for healthcare in Northern Ireland found that 47.73% of people reported that their health deteriorated while they were waiting. This most often related to increased pain and a negative impact on their mental health due to stress. Being on a waiting list also made people feel as though their life was on hold physically, financially and socially (Patient and Client Council 2018).

A study looking at patient satisfaction in an emergency department concluded that 'perceptions regarding waiting time, information delivery, and expressive quality predict overall patient satisfaction, but actual waiting times do not' (Thompson et al. 1996). This suggests that managing perceptions and expectations of waiting times may be equally important as decreasing actual time spent waiting for.

Recent research in pre-surgical interventions has started to show that improving health in the lead up to surgery can enhance recovery and facilitate a quicker return to baseline living (Carli et al. 2017). 'Prehabilitation', the process of enhancing an individual's functional capacity before scheduled surgery (Carli and Schneede-Bergdahl 2015),

P. Langdon et al. (Eds.): CWUAAT 2020, *Designing for Inclusion*, pp. 59–67, 2020.
https://doi.org/10.1007/978-3-030-43865-4_6

has recently been adopted into healthcare terminology with some hospitals piloting the services. An example is the 'PREPARE' programme which aims to 'train' patients for surgery by helping them with factors before and after their surgery such as physical activity, diet and psychological well-being (Imperial College Healthcare NHS Trust 2018)

A recent report by the Royal College of Anaesthetists (2019) claims that surgery creates a 'teachable moment' for patients to facilitate behaviour change that they might not otherwise embark upon. They suggest that patient engagement and behaviour change is a critical step in facilitating change. This shift towards patient engagement links closely with emerging trends in healthcare: (1) Patients are taking more interest in self-managing, wanting to be more empowered when it comes to their health (PWC 2019); (2) Mobile technology is positioned to have a huge impact on healthcare, making it cheaper.

With the available health information and mobile technology, patients are able to understand more about what to do for themselves. These approaches can provide a useful alternative for patients to take an active role in their own healthcare (Waller et al. 2015), while providing patients with credible information and strategies for improving their experience.

These provide the context for the study. To gain a thorough understanding of the experience of waiting for surgery, this study considers the experience of having an operation, from diagnosis to recovery, with the main focus on the waiting period. This was to understand the experience in a wider context and assess influencing factors such as expectations.

2 Methods

Therefore, it was decided to recruit participants who had undergone surgery in the past five years and could reflect on the experience retrospectively. Purposive sampling (Cresswell and Plano Clark 2011) was used. The sampling criteria included: (1) Over 18 s (2) Having had elective surgery (18-week pathway) within the last 5 years (3) Not classified as vulnerable.

Participants who had undergone surgery in the past five years and could reflect on the experience retrospectively were recruited via the researchers' network. They were emailed an information sheet before agreeing to participate in the study. They then signed an informed consent form, allowing for audio recording to take place. In Table 1, the participants' names were replaced with a code.

2.1 Data Collection

A visual timeline activity was used for participants to highlight key events during their experience of waiting for surgery. This provided a structure to map out their experience, while providing them with a visual reference to refer to during the interviews. The timeline was modelled on the tool 'a day in the life', which uncovers tacit and latent knowledge by encouraging storytelling through a layering approach (Sanders and Stappers 2012). This method was used to gain a detailed understanding of the entire process from the patient perspective.

Table 1. Participants' information

Participants	Surgery	Wait time
P1A	Triple Bypass Femorodistal Bypass R. Leg, L. Leg	Urgent Case 5 Months, 4 Months
P1B	n/a (spouse of P1A)	n/a
P2	Cervical Myopathy	5 Months
P3	Inguinal Hernia Repair, Hernia Repair	5 Months, 5 Months
P4	ACL reconstruction (Hamstring Graft) ACL reconstruction (Patella Tendon Graft)	5 Months 9 Months
P5	ACL reconstruction & Cartilage Repair Knee arthroscopic cartilage repair	4 Months 3 Months
P6	Inguinal Hernia Repair	5 Months
P7	ACL reconstruction	5 Months
P8	ACL reconstruction	5 Months

The participants were presented with an empty timeline split into three stages: before care, during care and after care. The aim of the activity was to understand three aspects: (1) What happened (the facts) (2) How they felt about it (3) Why they felt this way. First, participants were asked to fill in the events on the timeline as they happened to establish the facts. Second, they were asked to mark high and low points on the timeline by describing their emotions at each stage. They were then asked to talk through the timeline and explain why they felt the way they did at each point. This allowed participants to build a story and evaluate the individual experiences while being able to see the whole experience mapped out in front of them.

The timeline activity was followed by a semi-structured interview to provide 'personal accounts of experience, opinions, attitudes and perceptions' (Martin and Hannington 2012). This form of interview was used as it allows the researchers to modify questions based on participants' responses and probe any interesting or relevant areas that arise. Interviews were held face to face where possible. Questions were open ended to allow participants to influence the topic of conversation. The interviews were audio recorded and transcribed.

2.2 Data Analysis

Data was analysed from two perspectives. Firstly, it was analysed thematically using an affinity diagram to identify common themes. Second, it was analysed using a journey map to understand the data over time, in context.

Raw data from verbatim transcripts were systematically analysed and synthesised using an affinity diagram (Martin and Hannington 2012). Data were divided into individual meaning units and written onto sticky notes. These were then grouped into categories of related content. Each category was analysed to draw out broad findings to express the objective content. These were then interpreted to extract insights which expressed underlying meaning or latent content found across categories.

Journey mapping was used to visualise chronological actions and create narratives over time. It was phased in four stages along the horizontal axis: diagnose, wait, prepare, recover. The vertical axis represented actions, actors, what the patient is thinking, emotions, pain points, touch points, barriers and opportunities. Completed timelines were annotated with data from transcriptions. Sticky notes were used to record key pain-points and goals for each participant.

Verbal data from interviews were transcribed and analysed using an affinity map to produce five broad themes with 41 sub-themes, shown in Fig. 1.

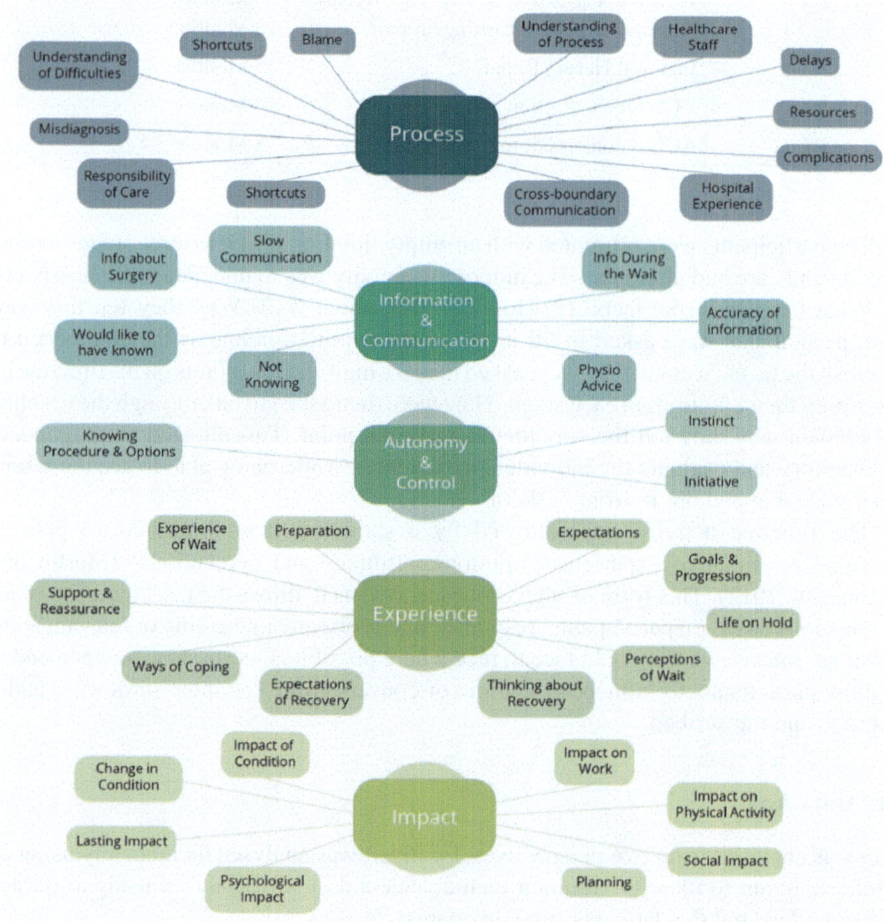

Fig. 1. Affinity map

3 Findings

The first theme related to the process that people follow in the lead up to an operation. Participants reported confusion at the early stages of the process and a lack of clarity of what it would entail:

"I think all they're thinking about is, 'We're going to treat your illness, your symptoms, whatever.' But 'Here's the process by which we're going to do that.' And 'here's who you need to speak to if there's a problem,' - that bit's missing." P1B

Additionally, people find it frustrating when healthcare professionals are unable to access their case information resulting in them having to explain their situation multiple times: "You'd kind of go and see one doctor and they would have absolutely no idea. You'd have to explain things to every person that you saw which is just really annoying." P5

The second theme reflects the information that people receive before their operation and during the wait. Participants explained that most of the information about surgery was received at the pre-operation, with very little communication during the wait:

"And between then and actually having the surgery, I had no communication at all from anyone. I just suddenly received a letter from them saying, 'Your surgery date is the. Whatever.' in the post." P7

"You don't hear from anyone for weeks on end and you just have to try and run your life while you're waiting." P8

The third theme reflects participants desire for autonomy and control over their situation. They showed initiative in taking an active part in the process by researching their conditions and their options:

"We did loads of research on surgeons in the UK specialising in knee surgery because it's an important joint to get right." P5

They also made decisions of their own accord, and sometimes persuaded healthcare professionals to change their minds:

"I managed to convince him to have another look." P5

The fourth theme centred around how people 'actually' experience the wait. Some participants reported overall positive experiences, and some negative ones.

There seemed to be a focus on the operation day, with less focus on the subsequent recovery:

"And also, when you've had the surgery, you're so invested in that's when you're going to be fixed, you kind of forget that for two or three weeks afterwards you are properly hobbling about and tired and grumpy." P1B

This lack of progression and feeling of waiting leads to people feeling as though their life is on hold:

"It was almost like you were put on hold, I suppose. Life was put on hold for a while." P7

People like to feel supported, and are reassured when they have sufficient information about their situation:

"I was desperate for someone to support me because by this point my physio had said, 'There's nothing more I can do until after the operation.'" P8

The fifth theme reflected the impact that waiting for surgery has on people's lives. In some cases, this was substantial, affecting their work and social lives. Participants

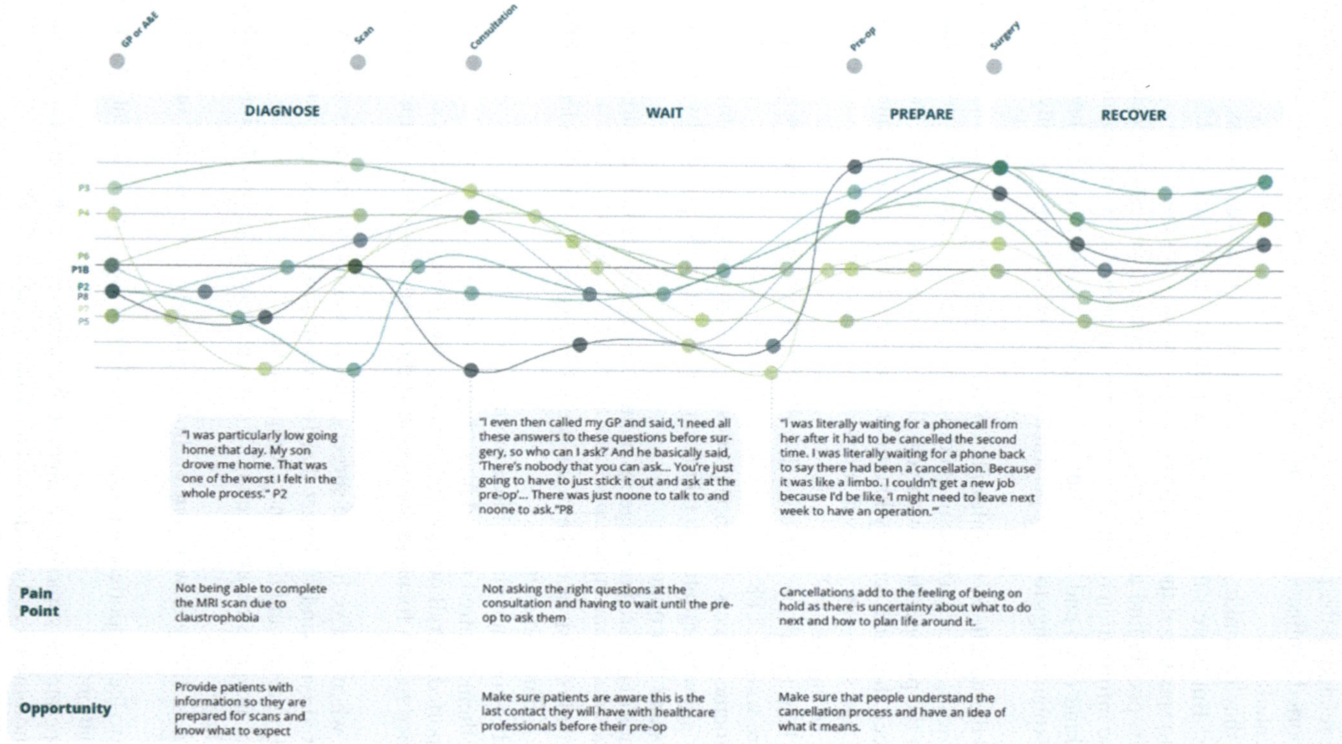

Fig. 2. Emotional experience

reported that their condition was always on their mind and something they worried about constantly, so as not to make it worse:

"I was wary of my knee at all times. I didn't want to damage it more." P7

"It sounds really pathetic, but there was a period where I just felt so anxious about if it was raining and if I was walking on uneven pavements because it just felt so unstable." P8

Anxiety was also experienced, such as fear of cancellation, loss of control over the situation:

"There was a lot of anxiety, hoping it wouldn't be cancelled." P3

"I had a bit of anxiety leading up to my second operation. I didn't even know I had it. I kept getting really panicky and I went to the doctors and they said it was anxiety about my operation." P4

Participants also reported that their situation left them feeling depressed, and this was added to by the feeling that no one really understood their situation:

"I'm not depressed. Not like proper depression, but I felt like no one really knew that it was affecting my life so much." P8

The emotional experience of each participant is shown in Fig. 2. Three key pain points are shown on the map that reflect opportunities for innovations to improve the waiting experience for patients.

The map identified key touchpoints where patients have appointments with healthcare professionals. These appointments are relatively limited in time and quantity due to a lack of resources in healthcare. This means that if something goes wrong or is cancelled, a substantial amount of time is added to the wait.

Additionally, these interactions may be their only chance to ask specialist questions. This means that if patients are unaware of this, or unprepared, they may leave without questions and have to wait several months to ask them at the pre-op. This can result in prolonged feelings of uncertainty, not knowing what is going to happen or how to plan life around surgery.

Finally, the wait after a cancellation caused anxiety as people had tended plan around their original surgery date. This was due to uncertainty as people would have to wait to be called in for a new date, leaving them feeling like they are in limbo.

4 Discussion and Conclusions

People Lack a Conceptual Model of the Process of Waiting for Surgery. This leads to anxiety due to fear of the unknown, fear of cancellation or something going wrong to making the wait longer. There is confusion about the process, and who to speak to if something goes wrong. Information they receive is not always accurate which causes more uncertainty.

People Want to Play an Active Role in Their Experience, Taking the Initiative. In the current process, the patient is passive, waiting for a letter to arrive telling them where to be and when. But people show interest and initiative in taking an active role in understanding and doing what they can. Additionally, people are experts in their own sensations, and instincts can tell them whether something is wrong with their body.

This is sometimes overridden by a medical professional as people respect and trust the specialist's knowledge and advice.

Low Resources Mean that the Few Interactions People Have with Healthcare Professionals are Crucial. Low resources (time and money) in healthcare result in medical staff having extremely limited time. People are underprepared for the small number of interactions they have with healthcare professionals. This leads to these interactions being less useful and efficient than they could be.

Life is on Hold Due to a Lack of Progression, Goals and the Ability to Plan a Future. People struggle to plan ahead due to not knowing when operation date will be, or in some cases how long their recovery will be. The only thing they can look forward to is their operation. This is in line with the finding by Sjöling et al. (2005), where the experience of waiting for surgery was described as "a life in 'no man's land' – waiting to return to a more normal life." While that study suggests that establishing trusting relationships with health-care representatives as well as having a sense of underlying support (from friends and family) can alleviate patients' distress, our study found that having a goal seemed to have a positive impact on the experience of waiting for surgery.

There are some limitations of the study: the sample is small, and the participants might not remember things in the exact way in which they happened and might be subject to hindsight bias. It was challenging to try to get the participants to draw facts relating to their emotions.

Health service reform initiatives have traditionally focused more on performance improvements and regulatory constraints, with patient experience receiving less attention (Bate and Robert 2006). This study has suggested directions for improving patients' experience of waiting for surgery.

References

Bate P, Robert G (2006) Experience based design: from redesigning the system around the patient to co-designing services with the patient. Qual Saf Healthc 15(5):307–310

Campbell D (2018) NHS operation waiting lists reach 10-year high at 4.3m patients. The Guardian, 13 July

Carli F, Gillis C, Scheede-Bergdahl C (2017) Promoting a culture of prehabilitation for the surgical cancer patient. Acta Oncol 56(2):128–133

Carli F, Schneede-Bergdahl C (2015) Prehabilitation to enhance perioperative care. Anesthesiol Clin 33(1):17–33

Carr T, Teucher U, Mann J, Casson A (2009) Waiting for surgery from the patient perspective. Psychol Res Behav Manag 2:107–119

Cresswell JW, Plano Clark VL (2011) Choosing a mixed methods design. In: Designing and conducting mixed methods research, vol 2, pp 53–106

Derrett S, Paul C, Morris JM (1999) Waiting for elective surgery: effects on health-related quality of life. Int J Qual Health Care 11(1):47–57

Imperial College Healthcare NHS Trust (2018) Imperial College Healthcare NHS Trust. www.imperial.nhs.uk/our-services/cancer-services/oesophago-gastric-cancer/prepare-programme. Accessed 3 Mar 2019

Martin B, Hannington B (2012) Universal methods of design. Rockport, Beverly
Patient and Client Council (2018) Our lived experiences of waiting for healthcare: people in Northern Ireland share their story. Patient and Client Council, Belfast, Northern Ireland, UK
Penin L (2018) An introduction to service design: designing the invisible. Bloomsbury, London
PWC (2019) mHealth. www.pwc.com/gx/en/industries/healthcare/emerging-trends-pwc-healthcare/mhealth.html. Accessed 19 June 2019
Robertson R, Appleby J, Evans H, Hemmings N (2019) Public satisfaction with the NHS and social care in 2018. The King's Fund, London
Royal College of Anaesthetists (2019) A teachable moment: delivering perioperative medicine in integrated care systems. Royal College of Anaesthetists, London, UK
Sanders L, Stappers PJ (2012) Convivial toolbox – generative research for the front end of design, 4th edn. BIS Publishers, Amsterdam
Sjöling RM, Agren RY, Olofsson N, Hellzén RO, Asplund RK (2005) Waiting for surgery; living a life on hold—a continuous struggle against a faceless system. Int J Nurs Stud 42(5):539–547
Smith JA (2008) Qualitative psychology: a practical guide to research methods. Sage, London
Thompson DA, Yarnold PR, Williams DR, Adams SL (1996) Effects of actual waiting time, perceived waiting time, information delivery, and expressive quality on patient satisfaction in the emergency department. Ann Emerg Med 28(6):657–665
Waller A, Forshaw K, Carey M, Robinson S, Kerridge R et al (2015) Optimizing patient preparation and surgical experience using eHealth technology. JMIR Med Inf 3(3):e29

Accessibility of Tactile Experience for the Textile Designer

M. Smyth(✉), C. Barber, and E. Zitkus

School of Art, Design and Architecture, University of Huddersfield, Huddersfield, UK
{marni.smyth,C.L.Barber,E.Zitkus}@hud.ac.uk

Abstract. The purpose of this paper is to explore the role of assistive technologies to support a tactile engagement in printed textiles that is accessible and equitable for all textile students and designers. The paper proposes that all textile students and designers require opportunities of access to tacit engagement and material sensibilities in printed textiles through equipping designer makers with relevant assistive devices for use in small-scale studio and workshop settings. This study reviews the literature and utilises a case study approach to address the issues that arise when a disabled design student puts into practice their learning in the textile print specialism. Through this it is demonstrated that as active players in society, disabled textile designers require equality of choice of both physical and digital processes, without predetermined perceptions leading to an assumptive use of one technology over the other. In response to debates concerning equity and equality and the impact of choice in society, the present study aims to share an individual's experiences and insights into the importance and relevance of practical and creative engagement in materials and processes in the print workshop while being disabled.

1 Introduction

Although technology use within the textiles industry is growing at a rapid pace, the use of traditional print techniques is still a popular choice even though more laborious and time consuming. When working with digital, you can get numerous designs and colour ways finished in a couple of days, but with screen print, you can spend one day just on one design in one colour way. When writing about screen printing, Perry (2011) stated "I could see the evidence of the time and energy poured into each print. I could feel the texture, the over prints, the accidents - the labor…There are things you just can't achieve with digital prints" (Perry 2011, p. 13).

With traditional techniques still proving popular, many Higher Education (HE) institutions offer this route, with a focus on screen print, with this being the case, it is imperative that these techniques are accessible to all so that disabled students have the same opportunities as their abled bodied peers. Treadaway (2016) passionately argues for the value of hand craft processes and skills that are specific to a textile designer and useful to bring what she terms "competency" to a textile design and "an understanding and sensitivity for balance, and composition". With universities having strong equality and diversity policies, reasonable accommodations are widely made, demonstrated by a post 1992 university document stating "The University is committed to fairness in

P. Langdon et al. (Eds.): CWUAAT 2020, *Designing for Inclusion*, pp. 68–76, 2020.
https://doi.org/10.1007/978-3-030-43865-4_7

its practices and in meeting the needs of our diverse student and staff bodies. Where appropriate and within our means, the University will take positive action to meet these commitments" (The University of Huddersfield 2016). However, as screen print is such a physically demanding technique, and the screen print machines extremely expensive and large in size, investing in an industry level screen print machine may not be a reasonable accommodation in this circumstance.

This paper will explore these topics by answering questions such as: Could the choice between digital and traditional techniques be decided due to the connection between the designer and their work? Could the designer have more pride in their hand-printed work due to it feeling more of an accomplishment? Is there an alternative way to invest in industry grade machinery to make screen printing accessible to disabled students? And, if so, how can low-technology devices be employed within HE institutions to support the practice of equity within the crafting of printed textiles?

1.1 What Is the Value of Maker Skills

The Crafts Council (2016) released a report detailing trends in provision and participation of courses relating to craft, with the research for this report conducted for the academic years 2007/08 to 2014/15. The report states that in higher education there has been a rapid decline in both craft courses and students. Between 2007/08 and 2014/15 HE courses declined by 50% in terms of undergraduate (UG) participation, however the report also states that, unlike other disciplines, textiles has shown a slight increase since 2012/13 (Crafts Council 2016). The research showed that 4% of craft-based students have a physical disability, nevertheless, the report did not go into specific details which craft courses this data applied to. This shows that, although many institutions offer courses in craft, it is a declining area of HE study.

The exact reason is unknown, however it could be questioned whether the rise in university fees could effect this. Another cause could be the rise of technology; many design companies now look to hire people with skills in computer-aided design, which can be learnt by watching videos on free sites such as YouTube. According to Lynch (2013) the traditional skills of drawing to scale and manual creativity are becoming obsolete. Although the author refers to architecture and building craft, the relevance of learning basic drawing skills raise a relevant point to textile education, specifically print. With the rise of technology, is the value of learning traditional techniques such as screen print lessening? Learning hands-on techniques such as screen printing not only potentially leads to employment, but also cross-disciplinary and community based opportunities. Robertson and Vinebaum (2016) discusses how galleries and other public domains are starting to run workshops etc. in traditional crafts for the public.

Maker spaces - prevalent in DIY, open source and hacker communities are 'popping up' in institutional environments in an effort to provide visitors with hands-on experiences of art making. Notably, the curation of *The Possible* in 2014 by David Wilson at the Berkeley Art Museum, reconfigured galleries into workspaces for ceramics, dyeing, printmaking and sound recording, involving collaborations between over 100 artists and members of the public (Robertson and Vinebaum 2016). However, when it comes to community, it is not just the general public that are important; Jefferies (2017) discusses how the textiles industry is one of collaboration and collective-making. It could be said that without learning traditional techniques, skills in collaboration will not be developed, as CAD is a tool that facilitates individual projects.

Treadaway (2015) investigates how the development of technology has positively impacted the printed textiles industry as it allows the designer to experiment and change designs without worrying about going too far as they can just “undo” anything they do not like. It also removes the need for a studio work space and printing equipment. Although Treadaway predominantly outlines the positives of digital design, the author also acknowledges the need for hands-on techniques. She explains how all the participants of her research interviews feel that working physically and with tactility while being able to manipulate fabrics, help with feelings of excitement over the designing process and promotes imaginative thinking.

Dissanayake (2000) discusses how in art people find pleasure in hands-on ways of doing things and also observes how technology can obstruct hands-on techniques. The seminal exhibition called *The Power of Making* also explores this, showcasing a curatorial rational that making by hand directly influences development in individuality and imagination (V&A 2011). Concomitantly, there is an element of having pride in your work. Magee’s (2014) research corroborates this, stating that job pride is positively impacted by spending extra time to completing a task successfully. Pride can then lead to designers feeling more inspired to continue creating.

In summary, learning ‘making skills’ in design increases imaginative thinking and is a value that designers give to what they are creating that can lead to more inspiration in the studio and workshop environment. It could be said that without learning traditional techniques, skills in collaboration will not be developed, as CAD used in print design is a tool that facilitates individual projects. Altogether these changes to students’ learning experiences will provide them, as future designers, with opportunities to reach their full potential.

2 A Case Study of a Textile Design Student and Researcher

This takes into account the researcher’s own experience of aspiring to work in the textiles sector and being physically disabled. The researcher’s disability means she is a full time electric wheelchair user and has very limited use of their arms, due to this she made the choice to take the digital printed textiles route as this was the only way she thought she could design independently and complete her undergraduate course in printed textiles successfully. When starting her Masters of Arts (MA), the researcher realised that she has a unique perspective on the physicality of designing. There is still a significant focus on traditional techniques such as lino, kinetic drawing, embroidery, heat setting and screen printing. The designer felt she had found some successful alternative methods for physically disabled designers, apart from screen printing (as shown in Fig. 1).

Screen printing is a traditional printing process whereby paint or dye is pulled through a silk screen with a print previously exposed on the stretched screen. This technique, although classed as traditional, is still widely used in education, in the printed textiles industry and is popular with small businesses and self-employed designers, for example Timorous Beasties recently hosting a commission of screen printed interior fabrics for Harewood House, Leeds (Beasties 2019). Screen print is very physical; arm strength

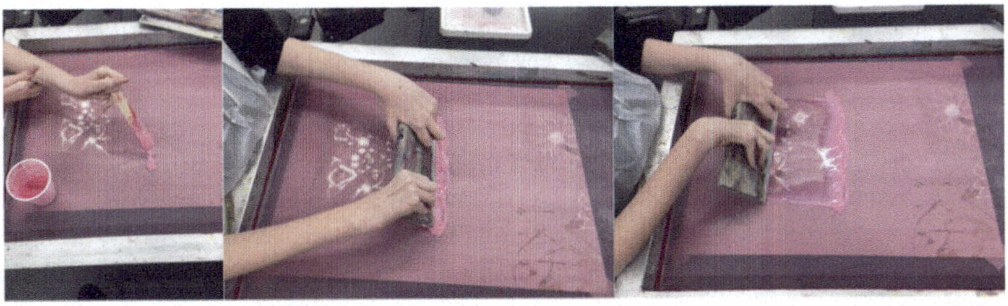

Fig. 1. Screen printing process demonstrating the sequence of the 'pull', as ink is forced through the mesh of a screen using a squeegee

and movement is needed as well as stamina. Although screen print machines could be employed, these are extremely expensive and space consuming - they may be an option for industry, but for disabled design students or self-employed designers this is not a realistic solution. The industrial machines also do not give the visual appearance that the manual manner of screen printing provides, with, for instance, miss-prints and mistakes sometimes leading to a designer developing their own unique aesthetic.

The researcher saw this as an equality issue, disabled designers/design students should have the same choice and opportunity as their able-bodied peers. This is why the researcher feels it is imperative that a low-tech assistive device is developed as an equitable solution so that disabled designers have the same options as non-disabled designers. The research project that provided the impetus for this paper, started with literature reviews on textiles and disability, progressing to inclusive design and terminology associated with disability, and life experience. It has, however, been found that the issue runs a lot deeper than simply designing a device. It comes down to knowledge about accessibility, technology, dispelling perceptions and understanding the difference between equality and equity. Quite often disabled people are offered equality as long as it meets cost/benefit protocols; this is an issue for both society in understanding that cost should not impact equal opportunities, but also for developers of assistive devices and the need to make them as affordable as possible.

3 Equality and Equity

Activist and human rights researcher Sun (2014) states that

> *"Equity and equality are two strategies we can use in an effort to produce fairness. Equity is giving everyone what they need to be successful. Equality is treating everyone the same."*

Equality is an important aspect of modern day society, without equality society cannot function to its utmost abilities. However, when it comes to disability, true equality has not yet been achieved.

Disabled people are of an unique minority as, at any moment, someone could become a part of the minority. It's proposed on Disabled World (2019) that

"People with disabilities are the largest minority group any person can join at any time, and due to accidents and old age eventually do. Disability will affect the lives of everyone during their life, it is time society changed to acknowledge this."

With this being the case, developing a more customisable and affordable way of designing assistive technology/devices (AT/D) would be a benefit to everyone.

Within the textile industry, two thirds of the workforce are over 40 (Williamson 2017). An ageing workforce means potentially more development of disability within the current staff, as well as aspiring designers who are disabled. A more inclusive industry would potentially lead to more job security and development for the ageing and disabled population within this sector. In order to achieve equality, it is necessary to make everything accessible. However there still is a notion of making everything as 'accessible as possible' and making everyone fit into one box. This leads back to the debate between equality and equity, Sun (2014) discusses the difference between the two, and the problems they can result:

"Equality aims to promote fairness, but it can only work if everyone starts from the same place and needs the same help. Equity appears unfair, but it actively moves everyone closer to success by levelling the playing field. But not everyone starts at the same place, and not everyone has the same needs."

This demonstrates how, without equity, equality can not be achieved. If equity was seen as a tool to achieve equality, full equality can be achieved. There could be perceived to be a negative association towards special adaption or special design. The para-athlete Hansen (2019) proposes that a wheelchair should be seen as a symbol of liberation and independence, rather than a symbol of disability. In this context, these assistive devices enhance user opportunities and abilities as well as positive user identity that can be obscured by assumption towards special adaption or special design.

3.1 Accessibility from the Perspective of Disabled People

Accessibility, or lack of, is constantly at the forefront of disabled peoples' minds. It is a constant worry and, although The Equality Act (2010) states access or reasonable accommodations must be in place, it is an on-going issue that does not seem to be improving. Then, when accessibility is talked about, it is often in regards to the built environment. Although the built environment is the major issue in terms of lack of accessibility, societal attitude towards access to assistive technology/devices are also imperative when considering accessibility. Bristow et al. (2009) define accessibility as "the ability of people to reach and participate in activities 'normal' to their society, and is a necessary condition of social inclusion and justice" (Bristow et al. 2009).

Using and understanding this definition means that there are a lot more elements to accessibility than just having step free access or providing a ramp. Once in the facility - is there a lift? Is there a lowered till so people can be served at seated height? Do labels, signs, menus have Braille? Are there signs for best hearing aid settings to use? Is there a fully accessible disabled toilet? Are there straws readily available? These are just some of the issues, in terms of the built environment, that need to be considered.

A factor in accessibility issues, is that quite often, disabled people are not included in the design process (Newell et al. 2006; Marshall et al. 2015; Zitkus et al. 2018). Straatemeier and Bertolini (2008) outline how accessibility can be used as a design tool for when developing policies, they explain that in order to do this successfully, there are several steps to follow. These steps highlight how it is integral that participants are used throughout the process in order to meet the needs of all (Straatemeier and Bertolini 2008).

Although their research was focused on transport and accessibility in general, not just disability, the points are still relevant. In order to make a fully inclusive environment, disabled people need to be included in the process, assumptions cannot be made and 'bare-minimum' accessibility should not be acceptable. Straatemeier and Bertolini's (2008) concepts support this, stating that "The idea behind this approach is to understand how planning for accessibility can succeed, one cannot limit oneself to the communication of scientific theories on accessibility – one has to test the use of concept in planning practice". This concept could be applied when developing new technologies.

3.2 The Role of Technology in Promoting Accessibility

The development of technology and virtual reality has made accessibility more readily achievable. Ali et al. (2013) state: "For many people, the use of technology offers opportunities to engage in activities that would otherwise be impossible. However, this potential can only be realised if the technology is designed so that it can support people in achieving their goals" (Ali et al. 2013). In fact, through technology some everyday tasks can potentially be more convenient for everyone. For example, online food shopping, online goods shopping, working remotely from home, conference calls for meetings, all make general life more convenient (Lavieri et al. 2018). Technologies can also make activities more accessible for disabled people to partake in, such as the work place as it gives the opportunity to work remotely (Lupton and Seymour 2000).

However, a misleading pathway would be to use technology as an excuse to not adapt, also it should not be assumed that every disabled person will be happy using the technology. An example of this is the Royal Pavilion in Brighton, where only the ground floor is currently accessible. However instead of looking at ways to make the second floor accessible, they recommend watching a YouTube video of the second floor, but do not make any concession on ticket prices to reflect that disabled people only receive half the experience. It is understood that it is difficult when it comes to historic and listed buildings, still places such as Castle Howard in York have managed to work around it and provide lift access. In this situation, a video of the second floor is classed as a reasonable adjustment, however it is a concern that with the growth of technology, this will be increasingly employed instead of adapting venues.

These assumptions could also be made in terms of accessibility for disabled designers. Although it is true that the development in technology has taken away some of the physical barriers for disabled designers, and that many designers do work in a purely digital way, the digital design options do not always give the same aesthetic as traditional hand-printing techniques such as screen printing. Misprints and accidental ghost printing can sometimes lead to the development of a multi-layered aesthetic that would not have been developed with digital design, as it was done by mistake. Quite often serendipitous misprinting leads to designers developing their own aesthetic and variations of techniques in order to achieve this design attribute. Disabled designers should have the same opportunities to explore and experiment with these techniques in order to develop this aesthetic. Moreover, it is not only aesthetic development that needs to be considered, but also monetary restrictions. Digital design software alone can be £500+ per year, let alone the digital printing devices and readily coated fabrics. There are screen print machines, however their cost is too much for many small-scale designer makers, while simultaneously highly space consuming. For design companies, these costs may be reasonable in terms of providing 'reasonable accommodations'. However, the same is not applicable to small companies, self-employed designers and design students, who cannot afford these accommodations.

It is believed that the availability of affordable AT/D would help shift societal views of disability thereby helping disabled people be as productive as those are not disabled. Access to AT/D would also help to prevent economic exclusion as it would support disabled people in gaining access to more job opportunities. This is the reason it is believed that developing a low-tech device for screen printing is critical. The device would provide disabled printed textile designers with an affordable device that would give them the choice of taking the digital, or the traditional route, rather than having to take the digital route in order to design independently.

3.3 Dispelling Misperception Before Designing AT/D

Another barrier to achieving full accessibility is negative beliefs about disability. Many disabled people can live a fulfilled life and achieve the same as those who are able-bodied as long as they receive the support and equipment necessary in order to achieve. Riley et al. (2008) covered this in their research, dispelling beliefs about disability as the first step to achieving accessibility and equality. This is shown in their framework which outlines the importance of dispelling misperceptions around disabled people, facility owners and staff developing collaborative relationships with their disabled consumers, developing solutions for any barriers, addressing specific needs of each individual disabled consumer, identifying the cost of removing the barriers and monitoring the on going needs in order to assure the solutions are effective (Riley et al. 2008). Although Riley et al.'s research is focused on fitness and recreational facilities, it is relevent to disability in general. The sooner misperceptions regarding disability are dispelled, the sooner equality and accessibility will be achieved.

An example of this in a gym setting is the Neuromuscular Centre (NMC) in Cheshire. NMC have gym equipment that has been adapted for electric wheelchair users, meaning they can do exercise as well as physiotherapy. This dispells many misperceptions that wheelchair users cannot use gym equipment, the researcher herself did not believe she could use the gym until discovering this centre. This demonstrates situations of technology existing, but it is just not readily available in gym settings. NMC is not a gym, you cannot turn up as use the machines as and when; rather you need to have a form of neuromuscular disease and be referred by a medical professional, you then get appointments to go.

It is imperative that knowledge around, and availability of, assistive technology is improved so that the misperceptions are dispelled across all vocations, activities and social situations. As a teenager applying to college courses, one college told the researcher that she would not be able to be a fashion designer as she could not use the foot pedal on a sewing machine. If the college tutor had more knowledge regarding assistive technology and had asked the college for funding for an automatic sewing machine, this situation may not have happened.

4 Conclusion

By considering past studies and a case-study based on a design researcher with disabilities, this paper presents the importance of physical devices and tactile experience when learning printed textile design. The paper recognises that technology has enhanced everyday life and that it can positively affect disabled people. In terms of printed textile design, technology allows for more efficient, precision designing that can be done remotely for clients all over the world, however there is a danger that an assumption could be made that all designers will be happy using technology. However, there are small businesses and self-employed designer-makers, who prefer to opt for more traditional, low-tech printing techniques rather than digital technologies, among them there are disabled designers. Thus, there is a danger of technology being used as alternative, thereby making solely the digital or virtual print-based techniques accessible and therefore preventing equality. Disabled people should be able to choose between virtual or physical, digital or tactile processes. Achieving equality is essential, but cannot be achieved without equity. Providing equitable solutions to access barriers will help to dispel misperceptions regarding disability, and therefore help towards changing the negative views of disability as it will demonstrate that, with the correct assistance, disabled people can achieve the same as their non-disabled peers.

References

Ali S, Al Balushi T, Al-Badi A (2013) Conceptualization approach for accessibility-aware framework. Commun IBIMA. Article ID 477923

Beasties T (2019) Useful/beautiful: why craft matters exhibition at Harewood House. www.timorousbeasties.com/project/usefulbeautiful-why-craft-matters-exhibition-at-harewood-house/. Accessed 17 Dec 2019

Bristow G, Farrington J, Shaw J, Richardson T (2009) Developing an evaluation for crosscutting policy goals: the accessibility policy assessment tool. Environ Plan A 41(1):48–62

Crafts Council (2016) Crafting professional practice through higher education. A collaborative PhD between King's College London and Crafts Council UK. www.craftscouncil.org.uk/articles/crafting-professional-practice-through-higher-education. Accessed 17 Dec 2019

Disabled World (2019) Disabled world – disability news and information. www.disabled-world.com. Accessed 17 Dec 2019

Dissanayake E (2000) Art and intimacy: how the arts began. University of Washington Press, McLellan Book, Seattle

Equality Act (2010) Equality Act 2010. UK Public General Acts. www.legislation.gov.uk/ukpga/2010/15/contents. Accessed 17 Dec 2019

Hansen R (2019) Rick Hansen Foundation. www.facebook.com/rickhansenfdn/posts/10155886927171470. Accessed 17 Dec 2019

Jefferies J (2017) Introduction: back to the future. TEXTILE Cloth Cult 16(1):2–7
Lavieri P, Dai Q, Bhat C (2018) Using virtual accessibility and physical accessibility as joint predictors of activity-travel behavior. Transp Res Part A 118:527–544
Lupton D, Seymour W (2000) Technology, selfhood and physical disability. Soc Sci Med 50(12):1851–1862
Lynch G (2013) Repositioning craft education and training to reconnect artisans to designers. APT Bull J Preserv Technol 44(2/3):3–13
Marshall R, Cook S, Mitchell V, Summerskill S, Haines V et al (2015) Design and evaluation: end users, user datasets and personas. Appl Ergon 46(Part B):311–317
Magee W (2014) Effects of gender and age on pride in work, and job satisfaction. J Happiness Stud 16(5):1091–1115
Newell AF, Carmichael A, Morgan M, Dickinson A (2006) The use of theatre in requirements gathering and usability studies. Interact Comput 18(5):996–1011
Perry M (2011) Pulled: a catalog of screen printing. Princeton Architectural Press, Hudson
Riley B, Rimmer J, Wang E, Schiller W (2008) A conceptual framework for improving the accessibility of fitness and recreation facilities for people with disabilities. J Phys Act Health 5(1):158–168
Robertson K, Vinebaum L (2016) Crafting community. TEXTILE Cloth Cult 14(1):2–13
Straatemeier T, Bertolini L (2008) Joint accessibility design framework developed with practitioners to integrate land use and transport planning in the Netherlands. Transp Res Rec J Transp Res Board 2077(1):1–8
Sun A (2014) Equality is not enough: what the classroom has taught me about justice. Mag Everyday Feminism. everydayfeminism.com/2014/09/equality-is-not-enough/. Accessed 17 Dec 2019
Treadaway C (2015) Digital crafting and crafting the digital. Des J 10(2):35–48
Treadaway C (2016) Crafting textiles in the digital age: printed textiles. In: Nimkulrat N et al (eds) Crafting in the digital age. Bloomsbury, London
The University of Huddersfield (2016) Equal opportunities and diversity policy. www.hud.ac.uk/media/policydocuments/Equal-Opportunities-And-Diversity-Policy.pdf. Accessed 17 Dec 2019
V&A (2011) Power of making. www.vam.ac.uk/content/articles/p/powerofmaking/. Accessed 17 Dec 2019
Williamson J (2017) UK textile industry sees production boom in 2017. The Manufacturer. Posted on 21 Dec 2017. www.themanufacturer.com/articles/uk-textile-industry-sees-production-boom-in-2017/. Accessed 17 Dec 2019
Zitkus E, Langdon P, Clarkson PJ (2018) Gradually including potential users: a tool to counter design exclusions. Appl Ergon 66:105–120

Designing Cognitive Interaction with Emerging Technologies

Introducing Activity Tracking in Healthcare Settings: The Merit of Self-reflection

M. Annemans[1(✉)], D. Van Dyck[2], and A. Heylighen[1]

[1] Department of Architecture, Research[X]Design, KU Leuven, Leuven, Belgium
{margo.annemans,ann.heylighen}@kuleuven.be
[2] Faculty of Medicine and Health Sciences, Department of Movement and Sport Sciences, Ghent University, Ghent, Belgium
Delfien.VanDyck@UGent.be

Abstract. To investigate how healthcare buildings, especially hospitals, need to be designed to take up an active role in patient mobilisation and as such contribute to patient recovery, we are in need of a research approach to map patients' physical activity in relation to the (indoor) built environment. Tracking participants' physical activity is an important part of this as it allows to collect objective data on the kind, duration and intensity of movement which can then be discussed in relation to the built environment. The use of activity trackers can thus be considered a relevant method as part of a larger research approach. We illustrate how self-reflection can add to set up activity tracking through registering with and experiencing of wearing an activity tracker (Axivity). To conclude advantages and limitations of the self-reflection process are discussed in relation to the complex context of healthcare settings.

1 Physical Activity (Tracking) in Healthcare Environments

Whereas people are admitted to a hospital or care facility with the intention to heal, or at least improve their (physical) condition, healthcare organisations continuously face the challenge of avoiding physical decline amongst patients, especially older ones (Boltz et al. 2012; Stall 2012). When the care focuses on treating acute illness, little time remains to assist patients in walking or performing other forms of exercise. Yet, keeping patients, with diverse physical and cognitive capacities, active – from early mobilisation after severe surgery (Santos et al. 2017), even in the intensive care unit (Sosnowski et al. 2015), to long-term rehabilitation (Sjöholm et al. 2014) – has proven to be crucial in preventing physical decline.

In an urban context, research in the field of Physical Activity and the Built Environment (PABE) has shown the importance of the built environment in encouraging people to be physically active (Chaudhury et al. 2012; Mahmood et al. 2012; Keegan et al. 2014). On the scale of buildings, the design of the built environment in relation to physical activity has only recently become a research topic. So far no studies have been found that objectively measure physical activity on a building scale, yet related literature suggests the value of expanding current methods in this direction (Sjöholm et al. 2014). Simply adopting methods from PABE studies is not obvious for various reasons like

P. Langdon et al. (Eds.): CWUAAT 2020, *Designing for Inclusion*, pp. 79–86, 2020.
https://doi.org/10.1007/978-3-030-43865-4_8

the divergent physical abilities of fragile participants and the according difference in mobility options (Annemans et al. 2019).

As the overall aim of our study is to investigate how to design healthcare buildings, especially hospitals, to take up an active role in patient mobilisation and as such contribute to patient recovery, we are in need of adapted methods that allow to map patients' physical activity in relation to the built environment. Tracking participants' physical activity is an important part of this as it allows to collect objective data on the kind, duration, and intensity of movement which can then be discussed in relation to the built environment. In this text we elaborate on the process of preparing fieldwork with activity trackers in a healthcare environment. Due to the novelty of the application only little knowledge is available on which tracker would be most suitable. Also lacking is software to process the registered data and present them in a visually understandable manner suitable for the desired research approach in which a quantitative data support qualitative research. Insight into the experience of wearing the tracker, especially in a healthcare context, does not seem to be available. We start by motivating our choice for the device, the programming language, and the way of wearing the tracker. We then elaborate on self-reflection as a technique to balance registering with how wearing the activity tracker is experienced. In conclusion, we discuss how self-reflection has added to setting up the use of the tracker and which limitations this entails.

2 Activity Tracking: Registering and Experiencing?

In the last decade the market has been flooded by wearables and phone apps that allow to track various activity parameters like number of steps, duration, or intensity, whether or not linked to certain locations. Setting up a study in which activity tracking is part of the research approach, implies deciding about which device to use. This decision can be made based on various requirements regarding functionality, feasibility, and desirability. Whereas some decisions were already made by the study design (e.g., no need for real-time output), many other aspects are still to be decided on.

An important issue to resolve is whether to opt for a widely available commercial device (such as Fitbit or AppleWatch) or for a device specifically designed for research purposes. Concerns regarding confidentiality of the data, exclusion of fragile participants due to reduced reliability and validity of data when not moving according to the accepted standard, and limited or no access to raw data (Breslin et al. 2019), made us choose a non-commercial device with open access to registered data (Fig. 1).

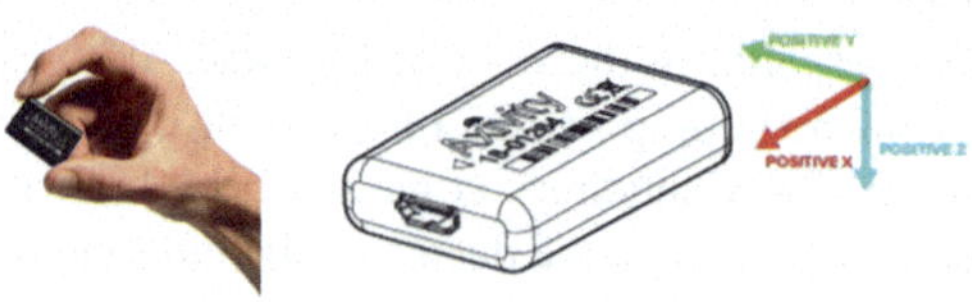

Fig. 1. Axivity AX3 (23 × 32.5 × 8.9 mm) (left) and axis alignment (right) ©www.axivity.com

According to these considerations we opted for the Axivity AX3, a 3-axis accelerometer with an internal memory and real time clock which allows to record data for prolonged periods (up to 14 days at 100 Hz). The device is suited for activity recognition and research in human movement science (Axivity 2015).

The producer of the trackers suggests wearing the device on the upper thigh or hip with the positive X pointing towards the ground. When wearing only one tracker at either place the focus lies on physical activity estimation (intensity, duration and frequency). Recent research has shown, however, that combining the data of two devices attached directly to thigh and lower back, allows to estimate physical activity and detect posture (sitting, standing, lying) (Duncan et al. 2018).

In a healthcare context, what is considered physical activity can vary significantly between participants and settings. Whereas at an intensive care unit sitting up can already be considered physical activity, in a rehabilitation context the intensity and duration of the activity may become more relevant. Therefore, it is important that the retrieved data allow to distinguish between different types and intensities of movement (walking, running, standing, sitting and lying). The programmed software should allow to visualise these differences in order to reflect on them in a dialogue between researcher and participant.

So far, the AX3 software (Omgui version 1.0.0.28) was used to configure the devices and download the logged data. Although an experienced eye can identify different bodily positions by interpreting the graphs generated by this software, this visualisation is nowhere near what could be used in dialogue with participants. Therefore, some additional programming on the data needs to be done. Since the AX3 is an open source device, we have substantial control over the configuration and processing of the data, yet the actual implementation of the programming requires a significant level of technological expertise and computer programming skills (Duncan et al. 2018). What exactly should be shown, which data are needed to be able to show this, and how these data can be registered through one or more devices has not been fully investigated but will need to be covered in a pilot study with participants in the field.

Given that patients in a healthcare setting often already find themselves in stressful and unfamiliar situations, we aim to limit the pressure put on them due to research participation. We thus pursue an approach in which they do not sacrifice comfort or feel restricted in their comings and goings. Therefore, we wanted to set up a research approach in which conscious programming allows to use as few trackers as possible, and the location and application of the trackers is closely considered based on the participating patients' bodily and mental comfort. The best way to gain insight into all of this and continuously make adaptations seemed to be to wear the trackers ourselves.

3 Self-reflection as a Technique to Set up Activity Tracking

Using the self as a starting point for research is not new. The term "autoethnography" has been used for various approaches to research in which self-reflection and writing are used to document and study personal experiences in order to understand cultural experience (Ellis 2004). Autoethnographers acknowledge how personal experience influences the research process and thus research outcomes and use the view from within as a strength rather than a weakness of the approach (Ellis et al. 2011). Usually the autoethnographer does not live through the experiences because of the research but rather recalls them in hindsight in function of the research aim (Freeman 2004).

Our use of self-reflection shows similarities but also important differences with how it would be used in a truly autoethnographic study. Similarly, the first author – henceforth the researcher - reflects on her personal experience, both bodily and mentally and regarding the development and use of technical skills and writes about this. Yet, rather than pursuing to understand cultural experience, we aimed solely at gaining first-hand insight into how it feels to wear the tracker, which physical and mental impact this has on the wearer, and how this can inform the choice for a type of tracker, the placement of the device, and the programming of the visual output.

Autoethnographic studies on the use of wearables tracking physical activity have recently been developed in the field of experiential computing (e.g., Prasopoulou 2017) and sport management (e.g., Baker et al. 2017). In these studies the authors reflect on wearing activity trackers and position their findings in relation to approaches and outcomes in their respective fields. In the former, Prasopoulou explores what reflection through memoires on the entanglement of data in daily lives can contribute to information systems research. In the latter, Baker and colleagues aim to show the benefits of collaborative self-study about wearable fitness technology and physical activity for sports management studies. These studies focus solely on how wearing the tracker and following up on the generated data is experienced. No reflective studies are found that focus on processing the data retrieved by the trackers, programming the (visual) representation of what is being measured, or technical opportunities for new measures based on the positioning of the trackers. Since decisions concerning these subjects are made in dialogue with the experience of wearing the tracker, it seems valuable to reflect on all of them.

4 Balancing Registering and Experiencing

Given that the research context and participants addressed are likely not the first audience the producers of the trackers had in mind, we wonder to what extent the trackers are suited to be used under the given circumstances. To start understanding the method from within, in line with the self-reflection technique, the researcher wore the trackers at different spots on her body starting with the thigh and hip as suggested by the Axivity guidelines and exploring new spots like the upper and lower back. During the 24 to 48 h periods of wearing the trackers she noted down any thoughts she had related to the research approach in general and to the trackers in particular. These thoughts could be anything from feelings of (dis)comfort, over concerns, to new ideas for the research set-up. Based on the researcher's reflections we illustrate the experience of wearing an activity tracker as a test for a research project. Our findings show how these reflections cover registering and experiencing, and diverse interactions between these.

Many thoughts are related to bodily (dis)comfort. How and where the tracker is applied seems to play an important role in this. As we aim for an application with the highest guarantee of uninterrupted wear and demanding as little effort as possible from participants and healthcare staff, we first opted to stick the tracker to the body with a waterproof plastic band-aid so it would not need to be removed when taking a shower.

To allow insight into what could be registered with one compared to two trackers, the researcher always registered through a combination of trackers worn at the same time on the thigh, hip, and upper or lower back. Some of these applications are more suitable to withhold than others. Notes about bodily experiences refer to how and where the tracker is applied:

> *"This feels sweaty, very greasy also, I really don't feel clean even though I just took a shower."*
>
> (09/03/2019, tracker worn between the shoulders with a plastic band-aid)

> *"Tracker on the hip: hurts! Putting on pants with a waistband at that spot is not a good idea when you are going to sit down a lot. Should I take it off?"*
>
> (08/03/2019, tracker worn on the hip with plastic band-aid)

These two thoughts illustrate that a combination of aspects defines how wearing the tracker is experienced. The tracker on the upper back is not only continuously being felt because of the location between the shoulder blades (both while moving as when lying down), apparently this is also a location sensitive to perspiration which adds even more to the feeling of discomfort and raises a continuous awareness of the tracker's presence. Whereas the location on the hip usually is not perceived as uncomfortable, this can be the case if one wears rather tight jeans when sitting. This highlights how unpredictable parameters (choice of clothes) can impact the wear of the tracker beyond our control.

Wearing an activity tracker also has a mental impact. Even a tracker that does not give you any real-time feedback about your activity level, like the ones you consciously decide on using, raises your sensitivity towards physical activity. Just by wearing the tracker you become curious "*how well you do*". As illustrated below this could influence people's behaviour.

> *"I almost forgot I am wearing this tracker today, let me quickly write down what I have done so far. This doesn't seem to be a very active day, I should go for a run tonight."*
>
> (21/05/2019, tracker worn on the lower back with paper band-aid)

Apart from the activity levels, being aware of the research aim made the researcher concerned about the research outcomes. This resulted in stubbornly leaving the tracker on despite feeling reluctance to wearing it any longer (as illustrated above) or in a raised awareness of how the trackers' presence relates to what can be registered and processed.

> *"Did I feel the tracker move? If it shifts a little the X-axis might not be vertical anymore. Will that affect the registered data? Or maybe it is a good thing, it will allow me to assess how exact the measures are."*
>
> (21/05/2019, tracker worn on the thigh, with paper band-aid)

Although why someone worries might differ between people, we can imagine participants being insecure about what is and is not allowed while wearing the tracker, whether they are active enough, or how they will be judged when the outcomes are discussed.

The combination of the above mentioned aspects defines how (long) participants are willing to wear the tracker (see Fig. 2). It also allows to compare the obtained results with the desired research outcome. By having experienced the wear first-hand, the researcher at least has a reference frame of at what point and why people could decide to quit participation. This is expected to help setting a realistic timeframe and weigh decisions regarding physical and mental comfort, optimal registration, and concessions towards the programming.

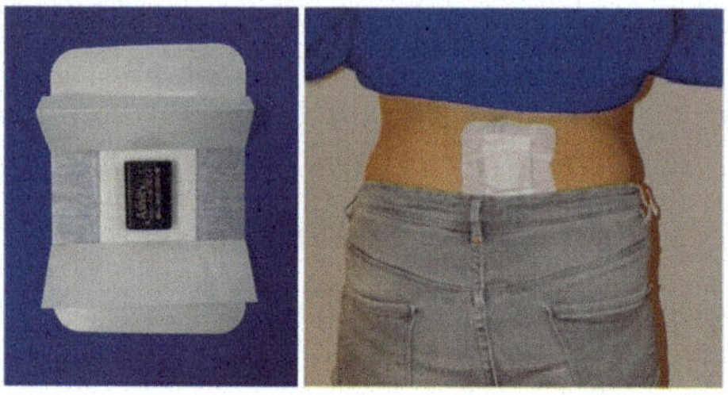

Fig. 2. Final positioning and application of the tracker

5 Discussion and Conclusion

As mentioned, activity tracking is a commonly used method to gain a good understanding of people's physical activity in relation to the built environment on an urban scale. Given the proven benefit of being physically active for patients, we wanted to explore how this method could be applied, or needed to be adapted to be applicable, in healthcare environments, being aware of the specificities of the population and setting. To be able to set up a research approach that is most suited for this context, without bothering patients with unnecessary preparatory testing we made use of self-reflection to gain insight into the experience of wearing the tracker. Additionally, the researcher reflected on how this experience relates to the process of working with the trackers (positioning, application) and registered data (programming). Whereas previous self-reflective studies on the use of activity trackers focussed on the experience of wearing and living with the tracker (Baker et al. 2017; Prasopoulou 2017), we considered it valuable to discuss this in relation to the experience of taking care of the registration. It is precisely this combination that defines how the research approach comes into being as a continuous dialogue between bodily, mental, and technical aspects. Below advantages and limitations related to each of these aspects are discussed.

The fact that the researcher has experienced wearing the tracker herself -has felt when it could be (un)comfortable, has been curious, and has worried about it- makes her not only more aware of issues future participants could face during the research but also provides a common ground to discuss these. This will hopefully benefit the broader research approach in which the (visualised) output of the trackers will be discussed with participants in order to gain a better understanding of the relation of physical activity and the built environment. This does not mean that the researcher's experience of wearing the tracker can be generalised. The researcher is not, and does not claim to be, a patient staying in a healthcare environment. Her experiences will thus be far from those of future participants. As such making use of self-reflection does not allow to develop a method specifically adapted to bodily difference like the way of moving, with a walker or in a wheelchair, or regarding diverse cognitive capacities. In this respect, the set-up of the research is clearly unfinished. Whereas at least a test with a wheelchair user is on the agenda, this one extra test will not be enough. It will be of key importance to approach each participant with an open mind-set and a continuous willingness to make adaptations to the method throughout the research process.

Apart from bodily and mental aspects also practical and technical decisions, play a role in how the activity trackers will be used in the research on patients' activity. Being aware of and meticulously documenting why and in which situation decisions are made, which can be considered part of self-reflection, helps not to lose sight of the broader context. Using self-reflection allows us to rapidly identify and react to possible technical problems resulting from adaptations made for experiential reasons. As far as we experienced, having the same person wear the tracker, know what she wants to get out of it, and be in charge of the programming, made her very motivated to stretch opportunities for adaptation to their limits to find a maybe not so obvious solution. A downside of this combination is that it requires quite some skills from one person. She experienced that it is very hard to ignore a personal preference for one part, and make the others subordinate to it. Additionally, being so closely involved with the aim and set-up op the research approach makes it almost impossible to judge how both process and outcome would be perceived by an outsider, which participants will be at the start of the research. Once again this will most probably ask for an extra round of adaptation once the research in the field starts.

With the study's overall aim in mind – to investigate how to design healthcare buildings, especially hospitals, to take up an active role in patient mobilisation and as such contribute to patient recovery – we started from the need for adapted methods that allow to map patients' physical activity in relation to the built environment. Self-reflection on tracking one's physical activity allows us to develop at least one part of a research approach aiming to do so. The combination of advantages and limitations of the self-reflection process to develop a tracking method, provides us with a nuanced understanding of what it means to do research and to participate in research with activity trackers. This seems especially valuable in a complex context as a healthcare setting.

Acknowledgments. This research received funding through a Postdoctoral Fellowship of the Research Foundation–Flanders (FWO).

References

Annemans M, Van Dyck D, Heylighen A (2019) Activating patients in healthcare buildings. In: ARCH19: building for better health, Trondheim, Norway, 12–13 June 2019

Axivity (2015) AX3 data sheet: 3-Axis logging accelerometer. axivity.com/files/resources/AX3_Data_Sheet.pdf. Accessed 18 Dec 2019

Baker BJ, Zhou X, Pizzo AD, Du J, Funk DC (2017) Collaborative self-study. Sport Manag Rev 20(1):114–127

Boltz M, Resnick B, Capezuti E, Shuluk J, Secic M (2012) Functional decline in hospitalized older adults. Geriatr Nurs 33(4):272–279

Breslin S, Shareck M, Fuller D (2019) Research ethics for mobile sensing device use by vulnerable populations. Soc Sci Med 232:50–57

Chaudhury H, Mahmood A, Michael YL, Campo M, Hay K (2012) The influence of neighborhood residential density, physical and social environments on older adults' physical activity. J Aging Stud 26(1):35–43

Duncan S, Stewart T, Mackay L, Neville J, Narayanan A et al (2018) Wear-time compliance with a dual-accelerometer system. Int J Environ Res Public Health 15(7):1296

Ellis C (2004) The ethnographic I: a methodological novel about autoethnography. AltaMira Press, Walnut Creek

Ellis C, Adams TE, Bochner AP (2011) Autoethnography. Hist Soc Res/Historische Sozialforschung 36(4(138)):273–290

Freeman M (2004) Data are everywhere. In: Daiute C, Lightfoot C (eds) Narrative analysis. Studying the development of individuals in society. Sage, Thousand Oaks

Keegan TH, Shariff-Marco S, Sangaramoorthy M, Koo J, Hertz A et al (2014) Neighborhood influences on recreational physical activity and survival after breast cancer. Cancer Causes Control 25(10):1295–1308

Mahmood A, Chaudhury H, Michael YL, Campo M, Hay K et al (2012) A photovoice documentation of the role of neighbourhood physical and social environments in older adults' physical activity. Soc Sci Med 74(8):1180–1192

Prasopoulou E (2017) A half-moon on my skin: a memoir on life with an activity tracker. Eur J Inf Syst 26(3):287–297

Santos PMR, Ricci NA, Suster ÉAB, Paisani DM, Chiavegato LD (2017) Effects of early mobilisation in patients after cardiac surgery. Physiotherapy 103(1):1–12

Sjöholm A, Skarin M, Churilov L, Nilsson M, Bernhardt J et al (2014) Sedentary behaviour and physical activity of people with stroke in rehabilitation hospitals. Stroke Res Treatment 2014:1–7

Sosnowski K, Lin F, Mitchell ML, White H (2015) Early rehabilitation in the intensive care unit: an integrative literature review. Aust Crit Care 28(4):216–225

Stall N (2012) Tackling immobility in hospitalized seniors. Can Med Assoc J 184(15):1666–1667

Preliminary Findings of a User Centered Design Study of Mobile Health Technology for Ghanaian Migrant Families

E. Owusu(✉) and J. Chakraborty

Towson University, Towson, MD, USA
{eowusu,jchakraborty}@towson.edu

Abstract. Mobile health technology has great potential to empower users and equip them with vital health management information. However, this potential is not fully realized if mobile health interventions are not based on end user needs and requirements. This paper details the results of an empirical study of Ghanaian migrant families and their perception of a tailored mobile health application. Specifically, the paper refines a prototype designed by understanding the cognitive interactive mechanisms of the targeted culture group. The aim of the project is to increase usability and adoption of mHealth applications by Ghanaian end users.

1 Introduction

Mobile health (m-health) technology offers great prospects in personal healthcare management and delivery systems globally (Chakraborty et al. 2018). The benefits of m-health intervention tools are correlated with the dissemination of relevant health information in a timely manner. While more users in developed countries have realised the potential to obtain personal health information to manage their health and adopt healthy lifestyle habits due to increasing health literacy (Sørensen et al. 2012), the same cannot be said for users in developing countries. Studies have shown that the use of mobile technology can largely benefit migrant families in the way that they manage their healthcare, communicate and educate themselves on public affairs and medical services (Wallis 2011; Owusu and Chakraborty 2019a, b). However, the potential to empower underserved communities is hindered by the lack of empirical studies and evidence-based research necessary to promote interest and adoption among migrant families. Limited research has considered the role of cognitive patterns of end users when designing mHealth interventions for migrant communities.

This paper reports the preliminary findings of a usability study of a prototype mobile health application developed through a user-centred design approach with emphasis on understanding the cognitive patterns of end users; in this instance, Ghanaians living in the United States. This is aimed at end-user inclusion at the requirement gathering and design phase of mHealth applications.

P. Langdon et al. (Eds.): CWUAAT 2020, *Designing for Inclusion*, pp. 87–96, 2020.
https://doi.org/10.1007/978-3-030-43865-4_9

2 Background

Before mHealth became a reality from a global prospective, the Ghanaian way of managing chronic diseases such as diabetes, high blood pressure, hypertension etc., and adopting healthily lifestyle habits, was largely dependent on visits to clinics and medical centers for information from medical practitioners. However, the advent of mobile health interventions has provided the platform for people from all walks of life to be empowered to be in charge of their personal health and lifestyle.

A preliminary contextual investigation found that there are limited studies on the adoption, usage and attitudes of migrant communities towards mobile health technologies. The focus of HCI research on human-centered technologies that are designed to fit the daily requirements of users is what is referred to as user-centered design. It is, therefore, important for researchers to be cognisant of standards and principles in the related disciplines, and always be aware of the target audience (Lazar et al. 2017).

Although the primary focus of user centered design is to collect data from participants of target communities, research has shown that limited focus on cultural diversity in the design process can affect usability (Chakraborty et al. 2017). The ever-expanding reach of mobile technology has ensured that users from diverse cultural backgrounds should be considered in the new matrix of usability requirement. The new eco-system of diverse user needs has created a cultural gap between designers and users. Although culture was a marginal issue in HCI, current studies indicate that culture has gained increased attention in mainstream HCI. This has resulted in the focus of HCI shifting towards a culture-centered design approach (Kamppuri 2006).

Culture plays a major role in cross-cultural usability. Reinecke and Bernstein (2013) summarised research studies that discuss the influence of user preferences and perceptions on designing interfaces. Language is one element that can affect where users focus their attention. For example, the writing and reading direction of a language can determine the way people design interfaces (Reinecke and Bernstein 2013). As a result, a single interface cannot be used to fit every user due to vast cultural differences. This calls for more research studies to evaluate HCI and understand how users interact with interfaces based on their cultural backgrounds. This is significant for cross cultural usability design to address migrant communities who have been sidelined in mHealth technology.

The importance of user centered design in the adoption of mobile health applications is further buttressed by McCurdie et al. 2012. They conducted case studies of user-centered design in the development of three mHealth applications that highlight the importance of usability testing of mobile health applications by targeted end users. Their study concluded that user-centered design is critical in the identification of key end user requirements that determine whether an app will be adopted by certain user groups.

3 Methodology

The main hypothesis of this study is that "usability affects user perception in mHealth". To address the hypothesis, a mobile health application was designed to better understand the Ghanaian migrant user experience. This study was conducted in several phases. The first phase was to identify specific user needs and requirements through a qualitative and quantitative data gathering procedure by means of questionnaires and focus group discussions. The second phase was to translate the user needs into a set of functional requirements and design guidelines by an open coding process. After development of the coding framework, relevant themes were derived and utilised in the design and development of the mobile application prototype called Motivational Fitness (MotiFit).

The prototype mHealth Application was built on the IOS platform using Adobe XD, Swift language and XCode. The process was undertaken with consideration of the conceptual framework of the Unified Theory of Acceptance and Use of Technology (UTAUT2) model by Venkatesh et al. 2012, which emphasises perceived usefulness, perceived ease of use, hedonic motivation, price value, and habit.

Using a use case scenario based on a previously undertaken user requirement gathering, a visual representation of the user interface was designed to form the fundamental structure of application. This initial concept of the application was designed by a rough sketch outlining the workflow of application demarcating the relevant features of the application, such as sign-up and login, onboarding, navigation, and menus. Sketches were then turned into wireframes detailing the design elements.

Using open user interface (UI) kits and wireframe kits in Adobe XD software, all icons and screens were then illustrated using ellipse, rectangles, pen tools, symbols and grids. More attention was given to the flow of the screen navigation layout with emphasis on the menu and the core features such as consistency and smart organisation, in order to reduce cognitive load and visual hierarchies. All screens were linked accordingly to relevant features such as Body Mass Index (BMI), food diary and workout.

Identifying the main screen features, the application was subsequently organised into screen functionalities such BMI, diary, nutrition and workouts, following the outlined workflow diagram. Below was the design process:

1. Reference to the wireframe already created was implemented serving as requirement needs for the application design.
2. An iPhone 8 artboard was created with the dimension weight and height of 375×812 pixel.
3. Placing emphasis on the Ghanaian national colors (Red, Gold and Green), the logo MotiFit was conceptualized and designed to fit the upper space of the application. The artboard background color was set with the fill tool.
4. A native UI kit was imported for IOS.
5. The screen layout was copied and duplicated for consistency.
6. Assets panel was used to make the design elements consistent. This includes colors, character styles, symbols and images.
7. General color scheme was customized to match the Ghanaian national colors.
8. Next, all elements were grouped, and each layer was named for easy traceability.
9. Finally, after designing all sections of the screens, the prototype transitions were linked according to the relevant screens. Options such as scroll and click were applied for easy navigation.
10. Changes made were previewed repetitively to prevent any unpredicted errors.

Screenshots of the user interface is shown below (Fig. 1):

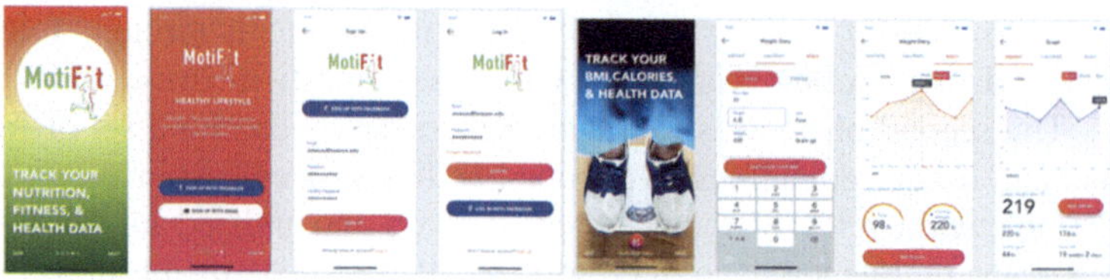

Fig. 1. Screens of the MotiFit application

3.1 Research Study

In order to refine the prototype application, we conducted a study using qualitative and quantitative data gathering methods to test an interactive prototype mobile health application called Motivational Fitness (MotiFit). The data collection was carried out over a three-month period. A questionnaire was developed with open-ended questions with free responses recorded using personal interviews, and closed questions using Likert scales. This testing study was important to validate the research problem of the study.

Research Question: Can usability impact user perception in mHealth?
After IRB permission was received, we began our study to answer the research question. A stratified random sampling approach was used in selecting participants comprising of Ghanaian migrants living in Maryland, U.S.A. Participants (Ghanaians) were chosen by word of mouth and recommendation from other participants who had volunteered. This usability testing included a cohort of 50 individuals in total. All participants agreed to have data collected on a one on one basis at a convenient location of their choice with no offer of compensation. Each survey lasted approximately 15 min. Data was mostly collected after work hours between 5pm to 9pm, Monday through Friday, and at weekends between 10am and 6pm. Participants were between ages 30 to 55. The purpose of the study was explained to all participants including the right to terminate their participation at any time. All participants were asked to sign a consent form. Participants were assured of confidentiality and no personal information was collected.

Each participant was asked to interact with the MotiFit prototype application on an IOS iPhone 8. Participants were presented with the mobile device with the application turned on. They were asked to look through and familiariase themselves with the application before proceeding to specific tasks. The mobile application task outline was then given to each participant to follow through. At the end of the task, the participants were asked to complete a questionnaire related to their user experience with the application. Below are the task list participants used in performing the task.

3.2 Procedure

Task No. and what to do:

1. Start application (Login) Preloaded
2. Skip registration
3. Navigate through the application
4. Explore the Interface of the application, taking note of colors, typeface (font) and layout
5. Explore the functionality of application example diary, workout and goals
6. Navigate to the BMI screen and choose Gender
7. Enter Age, Height and Weight
8. Calculate BMI
9. Navigate weight graph and recommendation to learn more about the BMI results
10. Exit and complete post-experiment questionnaire

Data was recorded by marking or writing responses on the questionnaire for the different question types into a excel spreadsheet. The IBM SPSS application was used to statistically analyse the data and examine the findings.

4 Results

In all, 44% of participants were males and 56% were females. 30% of participants were aged 46–50, 24% were aged 41–45, and the remaining age brackets 30–35, 36–40 and 51–55 represented by 20%, 16% and 10% respectively. Participants rated their knowledge of mobile applications as Above average (44%), Moderate (26%), and Technical (30%). 66% of participants strongly agreed that the prototype application was easy to use, 34% agreed. None of the participants disagreed or remained neutral. Despite the unique individual preferences and cultural pigeon-holes that influence the adoption of new technologies by indigenous groups, the results obtained in this study generally indicate a positive attitude towards the prototype mobile health application.

All participants interviewed had knowledge of mobile applications, with a cumulative of 74% indicating that they had above average or technical knowledge of mobile applications. This is very helpful in this study, as it indicates that participants are not new to mobile applications. Thus, their prior experiences, whether positive or negative, will inform their comments and recommendations to help circumvent mistakes of other developers and highlight key factors necessary to develop mobile applications that would satisfy the needs of the people it is being tailored for.

Descriptive findings were as follows:

- 66% of participants strongly agreed that the prototype application was easy to use, 34% agreed. None of the participants disagreed or remained neutral (Fig. 2).

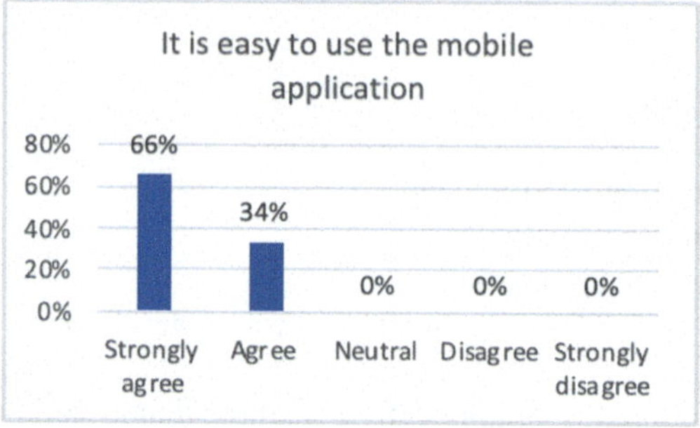

Fig. 2. Application ease of use

- 74% of participants strongly agreed they would use the mobile application if it was free, 24% agreed, and 2% remained neutral (Fig. 3).

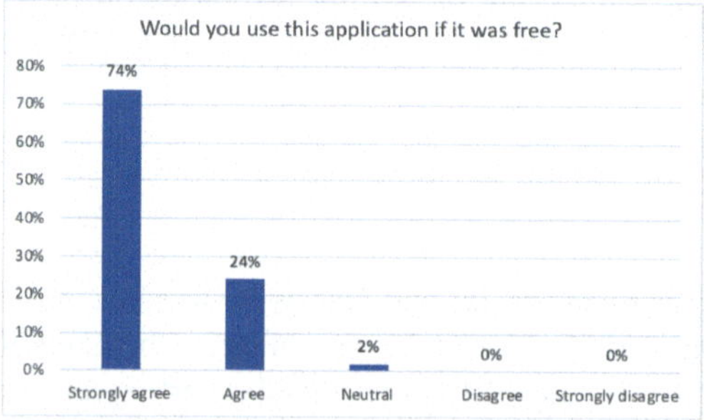

Fig. 3. Participants willingness to use the application for free

- If they had an application that could help themselves or a family member manage their health effectively, 62% of participants strongly agreed that they would use it, 36% agreed, and 2% remained neutral (Fig. 4).

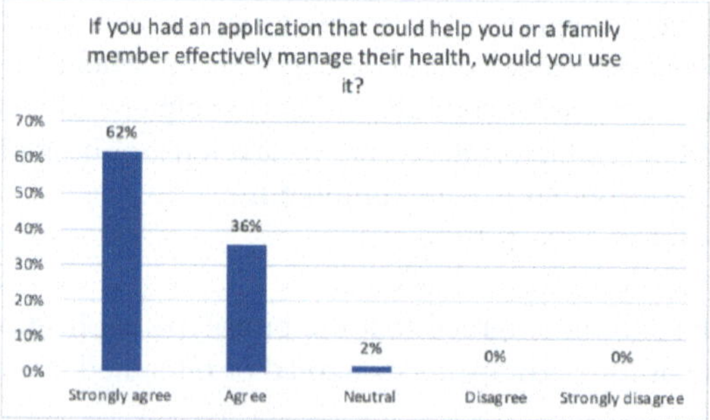

Fig. 4. Participants motivation to use the application to manage their health

- 70% of participants strongly agreed that they see personal benefits of using the mobile application to manage their health, 28% agreed, and 2% remained neutral (Fig. 5).

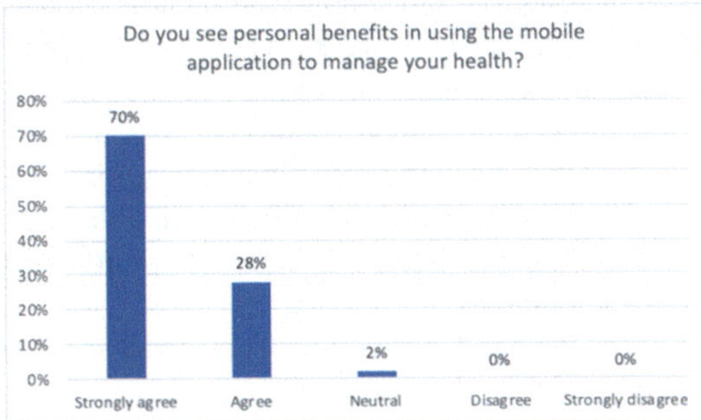

Fig. 5. Personal benefits for participants using the application

- 54% of participants strongly agreed that they were willing to pay for this particular mobile application if they knew it would potentially impact their health positively (Fig. 6).

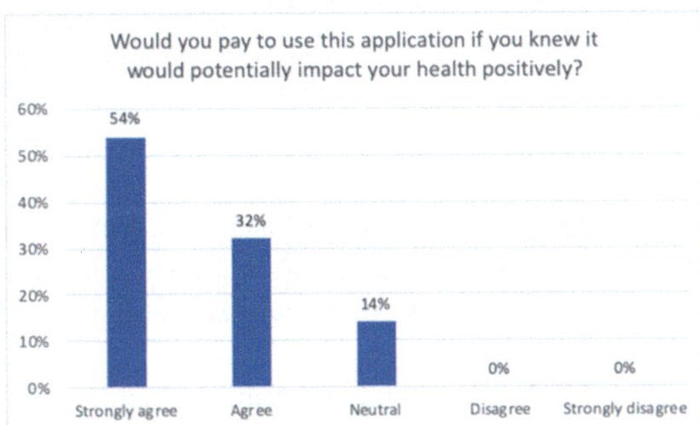

Fig. 6. Participants willingness to pay for the application

Participants indicated that the features they liked were the BMI (Body Mass Index) page with dietary guide recommendation, cultural features, interface design, easy navigation and ease of use.

Interesting comments and recommendations identified are discussed below:

- The dietary guide of traditional Ghanaian foods raised a lot of interest and most participants indicated that it was a feature they really liked.
- Some participants recommended that although the mobile application was being tailored for Ghanaians, in addition to the Ghanaian foods they wanted to be informed about other African foods in the dietary guide. This is a noteworthy recommendation as it would increase the versatility of the mobile application by making it appeal to migrants from other African countries.

- Others were of the view that they wanted to see more Ghanaian food categories in addition to those listed in the first version of the development. Interestingly, some participants indicated that they would like to also see other Ghanaian local drinks and alcoholic beverages in the dietary guide and recommendation pages.
- Older participants between ages 51–51 years recommended that the display should have a zoom-in feature on all pages especially for the dietary guide. They also expressed the need for bigger fonts and keyboard because of poor vision.
- Participants expressed that they liked the bold Ghanaian colors (red, yellow and green) used as a theme throughout the application but mentioned that the application should incorporate more of the Ghanaian "Adinkra" symbols (cultural symbols) signifying the traditional values of Ghanaians.
- Few raised concerns about the gender selection. They proposed that the section should include "others" as a part of the selection.
- There was a recommendation that the application should consider local or native Ghanaian languages as an option to be chosen in using the application.
- An interesting point to note, was the willingness of participants (84%) to pay for the mobile health application if they knew it would potentially affect their health positively. The willingness not only to adopt but to pay if necessary, indicates the urgent need of participants to be empowered to be in charge of their health. It also highlights the need to step outside the hype and to step up evidence-based research to prove the effectiveness of mobile health applications.

5 Discussion

The purpose of this study was to determine if usability impacts user perception in mHealth. Specifically, this experiment was established to determine if mobile health application user experience could affect Ghanaian end users to increase usability and adoption.

The results obtained highlight key social and cultural factors that need to be considered in the mobile application design process in order to engage, build and sustain the interest of this group of people (Ghanaian migrants) in mobile health applications. The willingness of participants to adopt and pay for a mobile health application if it met all their specific needs indicate that the usability of mobile health applications affects the perception of end users. This goes to answer the research question, however further studies are needed to substantiate these findings.

A limitation of the study was the convenience sampling method used, which could have resulted in the responses being biased. Also, due to the small sample size of the study, the findings should be interpreted as exploratory or hypothesis-generating, and further studies are necessary to verify these findings.

6 Conclusion

Participants in general held positive attitudes towards the mobile health application. The careful consideration and inclusion of the unique needs of Ghanaian end users during the design process cultivated a greater sense of ownership and acceptance as indicated by the willingness to pay for the application if necessary. End users are more likely to embrace mHealth technology when the implicit cultural values embedded in artifacts during the design stage reflect the values of end users (Leidner and Keyworth 2006). With respect to this, it is strongly recommended that user interface, user experience designers and researchers gain better understanding of targeted cultural preferences and the role it plays in the design process and usage of mHealth technology (Chakraborty et al. 2017). By developing a tailored mHealth application with cultural markers, it is envisaged that the health and wellbeing of marginalised groups, such as Ghanaian migrants can be improved.

Future research patterns should include expanding this study to encompass a larger cohort of participants from different locations. This research should also be extended to other migrant groups in the United States, to determine their perception and interaction with mHealth applications.

Current research primarily focuses on the different mHealth applications that are available, and their use for various health challenges, it is imperative that more evidence-based research is conducted on the actual impact of mHealth applications not just for migrant populations, but for the general population as a whole.

References

Chakraborty J, Chakraborty S, Dehlinger J, Hritz J (2017) Designing video games for the blind: results of an empirical study. Univ Access Inf Soc 16(3):809–818

Chakraborty J, Rosasco N, Dehlinger J, Wadhwaniya S, Tetali S et al (2018) Understanding cross-cultural requirements in mHealth design: findings of a usability study of Indian health professionals. In: Sezgin E et al (eds) Current and emerging mHealth technologies. Springer, Cham

Kamppuri M, Bednarik R, Tukiainen M (2006) The expanding focus of HCI: case culture. In: Proceedings of the 4th Nordic conference on human-computer interaction: changing roles, Oslo, Norway, October 2006

Lazar J, Feng JH, Hochheiser H (2017) Research methods in human-computer interaction. Morgan Kaufmann, Cambridge

Leidner DE, Kayworth T (2006) A review of culture in information systems research: toward a theory of information technology culture conflict. MIS Q 30(2):357–399

McCurdie T, Taneva S, Casselman M, Yeung M, McDaniel C et al (2012) mHealth consumer apps: the case for user-centered design. Biomed Instrum Technol 46(s2):49–56

Owusu E, Chakraborty J (2019a) User requirements gathering in mHealth: perspective from Ghanaian end users. In: Proceedings of the international conference on intelligent human systems integration. Springer, Cham

Owusu E, Chakraborty J (2019b) Usability impact of user perceptions in mHealth – the case of Ghanaian migrants. In: Proceedings of the international conference on intelligent human systems integration. Springer, Cham

Reinecke K, Bernstein A (2013) Knowing what a user likes: a design science approach to interfaces that automatically adapt to culture. MIS Q 37(2):427–453

Sørensen K, Van den Broucke S, Fullam J, Doyle G, Pelikan J et al (2012) Health literacy and public health: a systematic review and integration of definitions and models. BMC Public Health 12(1):80

Venkatesh V, Thong JY, Xu X (2012) Consumer acceptance and use of information technology: extending the unified theory of acceptance and use of technology. MIS Q 36(1):157–178
Wallis C (2011) Mobile phones without guarantees: the promises of technology and the contingencies of culture. New Media Soc 13(3):471–485

Designing Inclusive Architecture: Buildings and Spaces

Exploring with Children What Makes a City Child-Friendly

C. Ramioul[1(✉)], P. Tutenel[2], and A. Heylighen[2]

[1] Osar Architecten, Antwerp, Belgium
celine.ramioul@osar.be

[2] Department of Architecture, Research[x]Design, KU Leuven, Leuven, Belgium
{piet.tutenel,ann.heylighen}@kuleuven.be

Abstract. In light of the 30th birthday of the Convention on the Rights of the Child, we explore what makes a city child-friendly. This question is often answered by adults rather than children themselves. Moreover, designing child-specific places tends to bring children out of view. With an eye to designing cities as places for everyone, including children, we explored together with them how they experience their city. Findings suggest that they find physical boundaries exciting and are curious about what lies behind them; transitory zones (places passed through in the course of daily public life) are relevant to them in terms of independent mobility and affordances like play and social interaction; adults do not always see what places afford children and children themselves are not always aware of them. Societal challenges important for child-friendliness today include population aging, safety, and the environmental impact. Finally, children often do not seem to be aware that the physical environment can be improved, which is why participation remains important: it can teach children that they can do something about their environment. The fact that children have a different knowledge about the urban environment than adults, can only enrich participation processes.

1 Introduction

Since the implementation of the 1989 United Nations Convention on the Rights of the Child, the notion of child-friendliness has gained importance in Western society. Our study focuses on child-friendly cities: what exactly makes a city child-friendly? We make an attempt to answer this question from the child's perspective. Acknowledging the importance of working together with children when researching this topic, we set out to explore how they experience the city.

While children have as much right to the city as adults, spatial planners often make cars a priority and push children away to places that are specifically designed for them, such as playgrounds (Carroll et al. 2017). "No play" signs even ban children from playing somewhere (ibid.). Restricting children to child-specific places should make way for rethinking entire streets, squares, parks as places for both children and adults (ibid.). One way to integrate children further into urban society is to make more use of their participation in designing cities. This is also expected to improve design processes by imparting more creativity and a fresh perspective on design (Derr and Tarantini 2016).

P. Langdon et al. (Eds.): CWUAAT 2020, *Designing for Inclusion*, pp. 99–106, 2020.
https://doi.org/10.1007/978-3-030-43865-4_10

2 Theoretical Framework

To investigate children's encounter with the urban environment, researchers must go to places where children encounter the urban in their daily lives (Raittila 2012). Researching the experience of children requires respect for every child as a unique and valued user/expert of their world (Greene and Hogan 2005). Since 1989, a group of researchers who built on the 'new sociology of childhood' advocate attempts to restore the social outlook on children from biological humans in the making to social citizens and beings with rights (Bishop and Corkery 2017). In this 'rights-based approach', involving children is considered as the way to respond to their rights as citizens to participate in decision-making processes that affect their lives (Knowles-Yanez 2005).

Major obstacles of children and young people in all cultures – social and spatial – are connected to attitude. Social norms concerning children's value and acceptance determine the social processes of planning and design (Sanoff 2010). The built, physical environment is an expression of the society that built it; it is not only a physical but also a social phenomenon. Everything we do as members of a society is influenced by its culture and city planning is no exception (ibid.).

For our study, we started from existing concepts about space and place as a framework to get a grip on how children experience the city. Soja (1996) distinguishes between *Firstspace*, *Secondspace* and *Thirdspace*. The environment is understood as something that physically surrounds us and depends on people. It is material and sensorily perceptible and can be determined and measured empirically. This is what Soja calls the *Firstspace*.

The *Secondspace* takes shape when the material urban environment offers a variety of experiences or impressions. This also includes affordances, or action possibilities a space can offer someone (Withagen and Caljouw 2017; Gibson 1979). In an urban environment, a potential affordance can exist without the presence of children. Only when they enter it, it can be reinterpreted as a place where one can do something, like playing (cf. Rasmussen 2004). The experience of an environment cannot be seen separately from the person who lives in it. The place affects how a person experiences the world. The perceived environment determines the interpretation of life and our ability to act. The perception of the material environment (*Firstspace*) and action and interpretation of it (*Secondspace*) are inevitably linked. Children generate their own urban environment through their personal interpretation. However, their interpretations are not independent of the existing environment.

Finally, the *Thirdspace* (Soja 1996) includes the first two concepts, but is not just a combination of them. It also includes collective rules and values as well as the symbols of culture, politics and ideology. People (including children) who use a physical urban environment have cultural and social knowledge about it. Children know, to a certain extent, what it means to live in an urban environment and the public and hidden rules associated with it. They also have knowledge about using the urban environment, which can differ from how an adult uses it (Raittila 2012).

Oldenburg (1989) makes a different distinction using the concept of 'place'. The *first place* is the home, the *second place* the workplace for adults or the school for children. These places are clearly defined and limited to physical and social environments. By contrast the *third places* are accessible public places for informal public life, such as cafes, post offices and main streets (ibid.), public parks, or local shops such as restaurants, bakeries, hairdressers or small supermarkets (Gardner 2011). These places are important for children's autonomous mobility, social interaction, and development of an identity. Yet, due to planning or safety concerns, children are increasingly excluded from *third places*, despite their potential for play, physical activity, independence, exploration and socialisation (Carroll et al. 2015). *Third places* can be divided into destinations, specific locations within a neighbourhood, and semi-public places located between the private home and the public neighbourhood, such as porches, patios, back gardens and balconies (Gardner 2011).

Other, less obvious places are transitory zones (Gardner 2011), i.e., places passed during daily public life: the footpaths close to home, the metro platform, seats on buses or the queue at the counter in the supermarket. Being used as social places to interact with people, even if only for a while, they are considered especially important for older people and less for children and young people.

Third places and transitory zones ensure natural relationships and interactions; natural meaning "not forced" or "not formal", i.e., not with paid staff, volunteers, caretakers or family. These interactions are more universal (e.g., across age groups), often spontaneous, informal, daily meetings and relationships with non-family members (Gardner 2011). Destinations and transitory zones, in particular, belong to the domain of urban planning. The level of child-friendliness of such places can either facilitate or limit the use of public space, independent mobility, exploration and social interaction (ibid.).

3 Research with Children

Our study combined multiple methods: drawing, interviewing, walking and photography. Together with a group of 22 eight-year-olds, we tried to uncover how they experience their environment and what they think about their city. All children go to school, but not all children go to, e.g., a youth association. That is why we chose to do our research with children from a primary school, assuming that this group would be diverse. The school where we did our research is located at the edge of a city. The children were invited to make a drawing of the route they take to school, which then served as a reference point during interviews in groups of three. Subsequently we combined walking and photography. We took two walks around the neighbourhood of their school that they often take themselves (to the swimming pool and to another building of their school). The routes were chosen during the preparation of the walk, but the children were allowed to lead the researchers (cf. Cele 2006). During the walks, the children were invited to take pictures of what they thought was important. Both interviews and walks were audio-recorded, and recordings were transcribed verbatim.

Our analysis was informed by, amongst others, our knowledge of the literature and the theoretical framework, our collaboration with the children, and the *Zeitgeist*. We compared the drawings to identify common themes and elements, while trying to keep in mind that some elements are likely to occur less frequently as children do not encounter them on their way to school. We read the interview transcripts repeatedly to identify themes, both new ones and those already found in the drawings. In addition, we used word frequencies to get a better grip on the multitude of information, grouping words into different themes, each with their own colour, and using these to analyse the interview transcripts. Transcripts of the walking interviews and observational field notes were analysed using the themes already found and any new themes that came up. The photos were assigned one or more tags in relation to what is pictured. All photos were then grouped by theme. Also here, we tried to keep an open mind, so that potential new themes were not overlooked.

Finally, the findings of the drawings, interviews, walks and photos were placed side by side and linked to each other. After gathering all this information, the first author verified the findings in a class discussion with the children.

4 Exploring with Children

4.1 Firstspace

Nature is an important aspect for the health and well-being of children and adults (Freeman et al. 2015). However, children are increasingly excluded from these *third places* due to spatial planning or safety concerns (ibid.; Carroll et al. 2015). This is also apparent from our findings, since most of the parents do not allow their children to go out alone. Independent mobility is mainly situated in transitory zones, suggesting that these zones are also relevant for younger people – and not only for older people (see Gardner 2011). Moreover, the children in our study recognised in these zones many opportunities for playing, such as hills, walls, etc.

Sensory perceptions of a place contribute to people's orientation in the city, their understanding of spatial relationships and their experience of places and objects (Cele 2006). This became clear during the walks, as the children often touched things they passed by. Moreover, they were curious about things they could not see at first sight. Interestingly, the interviews suggest that children prefer peace and quiet, whereas adults mostly associate children with noise. During the study we also noticed that children often do not want to change their environment, or are not aware that it can be improved.

4.2 Secondspace

The *Firstspace* offers children many potential affordances (Gibson 1979), which are part of the *Secondspace*, and usually relate to play. When the children talked about play during the interviews and walks, they referred to two places with possibilities for playing (affordances): playgrounds and parks. These *third places* are important for children's independent mobility, social interaction and development of an identity. In addition, these places have potential for play, physical activity, independence, exploration and socialisation (Carroll et al. 2015). Children's enthusiasm when they see opportunities to play is huge. The fact that the children saw opportunities to play everywhere suggests that they interpret places in a way that may not have been intended by adults. However, children do not always realise this themselves. For example, they photographed each other while playing in places they know are intended for play (like playgrounds and parks). In other places, they did not photograph each other, although also there they started playing spontaneously (Fig. 1).

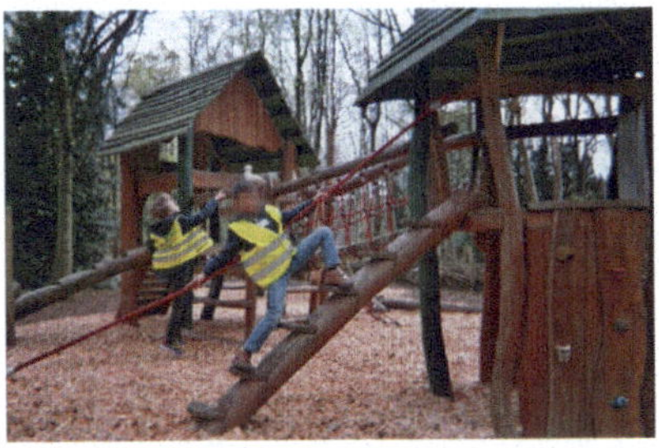

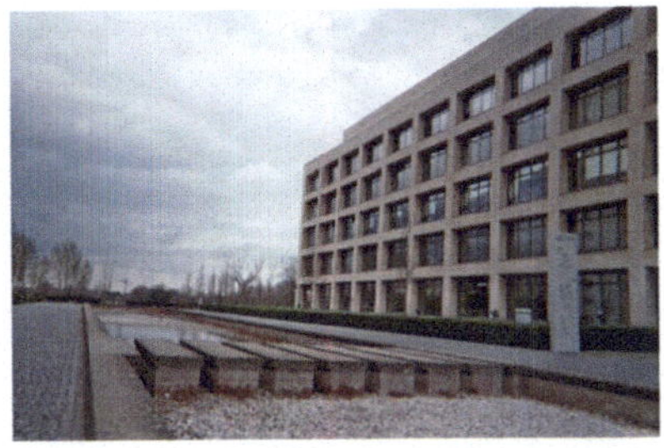

Fig. 1. Children find opportunities to play everywhere, even in places not intended as place to play. Left: a photo of them playing in a playground; right: a photo of a place where they also played, but do not include each other in the picture

Children are very aware of their environment. They showed interest in graffiti and art, but did draw the line with vandalism. For them the city should not be "clean". Especially fascinating for them is an environment that contributes to a pleasant sensory experience (*Firstspace*). For example, they find physical boundaries exciting and are curious about what lies behind them, as illustrated by pictures of a cat behind a window, or a police car behind a hedge (Fig. 2).

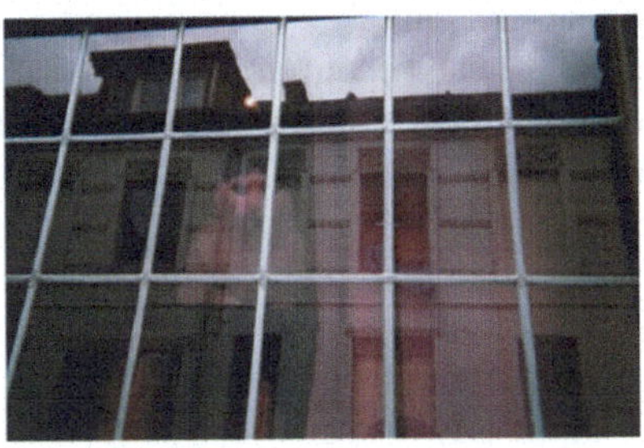

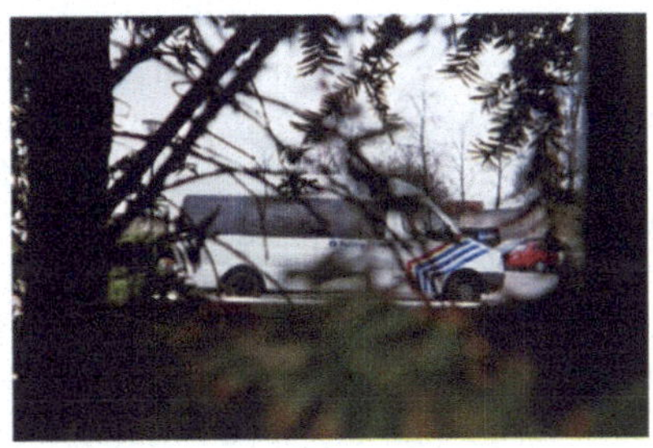

Fig. 2. Children are curious about what lies behind physical boundaries. Left: a photo of a cat behind a window; right: a photo of a police car behind a hedge

Most children indicate that they could find their own way in the city. The drawings suggest that they mainly rely on landmarks when thinking about their school routes, especially destinations (Fig. 3). These landmarks have a neutral meaning for them, but are important in wayfinding (Jansen-Osmann and Fuchs 2006). The children suggest that there are fine-space elements (ibid.) that could make it easier to find their way, such as a map, signposts with images, a GPS for everyone or electric signposts.

As mentioned, the physical environment is not only a physical but also a social phenomenon (Sanoff 2010). In our study, social interaction relates primarily to people or animals the children encounter along the way. Children find it interesting to interact with strangers because it can lead to new friendships. However, they find interaction with people they know more pleasant. Children also paid much attention to animals, often noticing insects or other animals that the researchers did not. Interviews suggest that children see animals as potential friends and also interact with them.

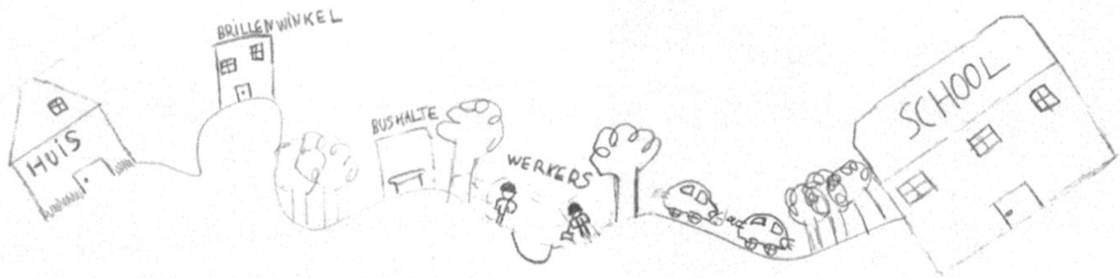

Fig. 3. Drawing showing that children rely on landmarks to recall their school route

4.3 Thirdspace

Children have knowledge about using the urban environment, e.g., they are well aware of traffic rules. These collective rules and values, which are part of the *Thirdspace*, seem to be inherited mainly from their parents. Children know, to a certain extent, what it means to live in an urban environment and the public and hidden rules associated with it. They also have knowledge about how to use the urban environment, which may differ from how an adult uses it (Raittila 2012).

Many children turned out to be concerned with environmental impact, climate change and global warming. One reason for this could be the current *Zeitgeist*, and recent climate demonstrations. Children's knowledge about this can also be associated with the *Thirdspace*. Children have a good knowledge of what can benefit (trees, cycle paths) or harm (CO2 emissions, waste) the environment. They even suggested solutions to improve the environment and reminded each other when they were doing things that could have a negative impact.

The difference in *Thirdspace* between parents and children could be a reason why most children are not allowed to walk on their own by their parents and are restricted in their freedom (Freeman et al. 2015). However, most children who participated in our study indicate that they could find their own way in the city. Our findings suggest that the busy traffic causes a feeling of insecurity in children and reduces their wayfinding capacities. This feeling of insecurity about traffic is heightened by concerns of their parents (Christensen and O'Brien 2003). Other research suggests that social limitations (imposed by society and parents) can cause a reduction in independent mobility, which has an impact on children's freedom (Freeman et al. 2015).

5 Discussion and Conclusion

Our study suggests that adults do not always see what places afford children. Children find physical boundaries exciting and are curious about what lies behind them. The fact that children see opportunities to play everywhere, suggests that they interpret places in a way that might not have been anticipated (by adults). However, children do not always realise this themselves; e.g., they did take pictures of play in places specifically intended for it, but not in places where they started playing spontaneously.

Much-used in new urban projects that intend to take children into account are "play and move stimuli". Urban planners use these to indicate that they incorporate small interventions which can stimulate children to play and move (e.g., steppingstones, little walls, fountains). However, our study suggests that for children the physical environment offers such affordances everywhere. This raises the question whether adults should determine for children where they should play with these play and move stimuli. Since our findings suggest that children are very well capable of seeing affordances for play or social interaction, these stimuli may be more of an addition. They are an interesting topic for further research.

According to Gardner (2011), transitory zones are especially important for older people and less for children and young people. The fact that these zones are important for the social interaction of older people might explain why tensions exist between younger and older people in public space (e.g., loitering youth). However, our study suggests that these zones are also relevant for children – in terms of independent mobility and affordances such as play and social interaction. If cities are adapted for children, people with an impairment or older people may also benefit. This is in line with the principle "what is good for children is good for everyone" (UNICEF 2018).

Besides aging and rejuvenation, another societal challenge is safety. Parents often restrict their children in moving alone through *third places* because of road safety and "stranger danger". However, social limitations (from parents and society) reduce independent mobility, which impacts on children's freedom (Freeman et al. 2015). Children have knowledge about how to use the urban environment (*Thirdspace*), which can differ from how an adult uses it (Soja 1996). Children may be more careful when moving around the city without their parents.

Based on our study we can add another challenge: environmental impact. Many children turned out to be concerned with the environment, climate and global warming. By taking this into account, they think of their future.

Finally, during the study we noticed that children often do not want to change their physical environment, or are not aware that it can be improved. They could gain experience with this through participation processes, evolving from a consultative to a collaborative or even a child and youth-led approach (UNICEF 2018). The knowledge children have about how to use the urban environment can differ from how an adult uses it. Acknowledging this can only enrich participation processes.

References

Bishop K, Corkery L (2017) Designing cities with children and young people. Routledge, New York

Carroll P, Witten K, Kearns R, Donovan P (2015) Kids in the city. J Urban Des 20(4):417–436

Carroll P, Witten K, Stewart C (2017) Children are citizens too. Built Environ 43(2):272–289

Cele S (2006) Communicating place. PhD thesis, Stockholm University, Stockholm, Sweden

Christensen P, O'Brien M (eds) (2003) Children in the city: home, neighbourhood and community. Routledge Falmer, New York and Taylor & Francis Group, London

Derr V, Tarantini E (2016) Because we are all people. Local Environ 21(12):1534–1556

Freeman C, Van Heezik Y, Hand K, Stein A (2015) Making cities more child- and nature- friendly. Children Youth Environ 25(2):176–207

Gardner PJ (2011) Natural neighbourhood networks. J Aging Stud 25(3):263–271

Gibson JJ (1979) The ecological approach to visual perception. Houghton Mifflin and Company, Boston

Greene S, Hogan D (eds) (2005) Researching children's experience: methods and approaches. Sage, London
Jansen-Osmann P, Fuchs P (2006) Wayfinding behavior and spatial knowledge of adults and children in a virtual environment. Exp Psychol 53(3):171–181
Knowles-Yanez K (2005) Children's participation in planning processes. J Plan Lit 20(1):3–14
Oldenburg R (1989) The great good place: cafes, coffee shops, bookstores, bars, hair salons, and other hangouts at the heart of a community. Paragon House, New York
Raittila R (2012) With children in their lived place. Int J Early Years Educ 20(3):270–279
Rasmussen K (2004) Places for children – Children's places. Childhood 11(2):155–173
Sanoff H (2010) Community participation methods in design and planning. Wiley, Hoboken
Soja EW (1996) Thirdspace: journeys to Los Angeles and other real-and-imagined places. Blackwell, Oxford
UNICEF (2018) Child friendly cities and communities handbook. www.unicef.org/eap/reports/child-friendly-cities-and-communities-handbook. Accessed 19 Dec 2019
Withagen R, Caljouw SR (2017) Aldo van Eyck's playgrounds. Front Psychol 8:1130

Reflections on Methods for Exploring Children's Encounter with the Urban Environment

C. Ramioul[1(✉)], P. Tutenel[2], and A. Heylighen[2]

[1] Osar Architecten, Antwerp, Belgium
celine.ramioul@osar.be
[2] Department of Architecture, Research[x]Design, KU Leuven, Leuven, Belgium
{piet.tutenel,ann.heylighen}@kuleuven.be

Abstract. While children have as much right to the city as other people, spatial planners tend to restrict them to child-specific places such as playgrounds. With an eye to designing cities as places for everyone, we explored together with children how they experience their city and what they think about it. In this paper we reflect on the use of research methods in our exploration. In our attempt to engage a group of 22 eight-year-olds, we used a combination of drawing, interviewing, walking and photography. Findings and feedback from the children teach us that they interpret things in their own distinctive way, highlighting the importance of involving them in research and other processes from start to end. Moreover, whereas participation is usually set up with an eye to future changes, our study shows the value of studying how children see and do things in its own right.

1 Introduction

Children have as much right to the city as other people. Nevertheless, spatial planners often push children away to places that are specifically designed for them, such as playgrounds (Carroll et al. 2017; Carroll et al. 2019). "No play" signs even ban children from playing in specific places. If cities are to be designed inclusively, restricting children to child-specific places should make way for rethinking entire streets, squares, parks as places for everyone, including children.

Our research focuses on child-friendly cities: what exactly makes a city child-friendly? We make an attempt to answer this question from the child's perspective. Acknowledging the importance of working together with children in this endeavour, we set out to explore how they experience the city. In this paper we describe and reflect on methodological challenges we ran into when exploring children's encounter with the urban environment, and lessons learned that may be relevant for involving children in future research and policymaking.

2 Research with Children

Researching the experience of children requires respect for every child as a unique and valued user/expert of his or her world (Greene and Hogan 2005). Since 1989, a group of researchers who built on the 'new sociology of childhood' advocate attempts to reframe

P. Langdon et al. (Eds.): CWUAAT 2020, *Designing for Inclusion*, pp. 107–114, 2020.
https://doi.org/10.1007/978-3-030-43865-4_11

the social outlook on children from 'biological humans in the making' to social 'citizens and creatures with rights' (Bishop and Corkery 2017). In this 'rights-based approach', involving children is considered as the way to respond to their rights as citizens to participate in decision-making processes that affect their lives (Knowles-Yanez 2005).

Genuinely involving children requires using research methods that support verbal and non-verbal expression of lived experiences, are close to the lived world and possibilities of children, and recognise their uniqueness and diversity (Dedding et al. 2013; Hackett et al. 2015). Therefore, all methods should be participative and nondirective and enable participants to share control and ownership of the generated materials (Procter and Hatton 2015).

Moreover, researching children's encounter with the urban environment requires researchers to go to places where children encounter the urban in their daily lives (Raittila 2012). How children experience space is multidimensional, involving both concrete experiences and abstract processes (Cele 2006). In this paper, 'concrete experiences of a space' refers to sensory experiences and affordances (action-possibilities that a space offers someone) (Withagen and Caljouw 2017; Gibson 1979), while 'abstract processes' refers to giving meaning to a space. Different methods reveal different aspects of these dimensions: the methods creative and interactive aspects, and how they reflect power relations, affect how and what children communicate.

A first set of methods which are found to be successful in research with children concerns visual methods like drawing (Elden 2013). They offer a route to understanding children in other than solely verbal ways. Without an appreciation of the role of non-verbal modes in children's practices, there is a risk of underestimating the complexity of these practices and of defining children in terms of what they do not do, rather than what they do.

Drawing in particular is often part of their daily lives, tends to be experienced as pleasant and relaxing, and can, amongst others, help to remember things or turn something abstract into something concrete (ibid.). It can provide children with ways to record and reflect on aspects of their lives and generate multidimensional data. Because drawing does not require interaction with a space or with the researcher, the motives of the drawings can be influenced by previous experiences and context, which suggests that the child's processes of giving meaning to something are very important (Mitchell 2006). Because of their emotional meanings, drawings are more a projection than a reproduction (Cele 2006).

Another visual and creative research method is photography, which – unlike drawing – is place-interactive. While the photos contain both sensory aspects of and meanings given to the place, taking photos appears to be the most successful method for children to express the meanings they attribute to their place experiences (Cele 2006). Photographs of things, places and people in their neighbourhood give an indication of what they find important (Rasmussen and Smidt 2003). Once photos are taken, they can act as a tangible representation of the children's interests, allowing researchers to return to a topic for further discussion with them. Since children have taken the photos themselves, their interest might stimulate a discussion (Cook and Hess 2007).

Besides as research material in themselves, drawings or photos children make can be interesting in combination with interviews. Using drawings/photos as reference points to start an interview from, makes children more involved in the interview, ensuring a more informal conversation and settlement of the asymmetrical power relations (Rasmussen and Smidt 2003).

Interesting about 'walking interviews' is that they bring together the verbal and the sensory (Coemans et al. 2018). Explicit exposure to environmental factors may stimulate participants to answer, making them less inclined to guess at what is the 'correct' or expected answer to give (Coemans et al. 2018).

Walking is a method that ensures interaction both with a place and between participants (Cele 2006). Children are often very enthusiastic about the fact that they can go outside during school hours. A walk can also include 'unimportant places', like routes that children often use, but would not come up in sedentary interviews. A walk in an environment that is familiar also creates a different kind of relationship, since the children have more knowledge about their environment and can therefore take charge of the situation. Researchers may either ask children to guide them to their important places or determine the routes in advance, but still allow the children to lead them and sometimes deviate from the route.

3 Our Approach

Our study combined several of the abovementioned methods: drawing, interviewing, walking and photography. Together with a group of 22 eight-year-olds, we tried to uncover how they experience their city and what they think about it. All children go to school, but not all children go to e.g., a youth assocation. That is why we chose to do our research with children from a primary school, assuming that this group would be diverse. The school where we did our research is located at the edge of a city. The children were invited to make a drawing of the route they take to school, which then served as a reference point during interviews in groups of three. Subsequently, we combined walking and photography. In the neighbourhood of their school the first and second author took two walks that they often take themselves (to the swimming pool and to another building of their school). During the walks, the children were invited to take photos of what they thought was important. Both interviews and walks were audio-recorded, and recordings were transcribed verbatim. The resulting materials were placed side by side and linked to each other, after which the first author verified preliminary findings in a class discussion with the children.

Our analysis was informed by, amongst others, our knowledge of the literature and the conceptual framework (see Table 1), our collaboration with the children, and the Zeitgeist. To understand how children experience the city, we started from existing concepts about space and place by Soja (1996), Oldenburg (1989), and Gardner (2011), combined with the abovementioned distinction between concrete experiences and abstract processes.

Table 1. Conceptual framework

<table>
<tr><th>Soja</th><th>Meaning</th><th>Oldenburg</th><th>Meaning</th><th>Gardner</th><th>Meaning</th></tr>
<tr><td rowspan="5">Firstspace</td><td rowspan="5">– Physical environment
– Sensory perceptible (concrete Cele)</td><td>First place</td><td>Home</td><td rowspan="2" colspan="2"></td></tr>
<tr><td>Second place</td><td>Work</td></tr>
<tr><td rowspan="2">Third place</td><td rowspan="2">Public places</td><td>Destinations</td><td>Specific locations</td></tr>
<tr><td>Thresholds</td><td>Semi-public places</td></tr>
<tr><td colspan="2"></td><td>Transitory zones</td><td>Places passed by in daily life</td></tr>
<tr><td>Secondspace</td><td>– Experiences or impressions of the Firstspace (abstract Cele)
– Affordances (Gibson) (concrete Cele)</td><td></td><td></td><td></td><td></td></tr>
<tr><td>Thirdspace</td><td>– Collective rules and values
– Cultural and social background</td><td></td><td></td><td></td><td></td></tr>
</table>

To get a grip on all the different materials we gathered (drawings, transcripts of interviews and walks, photos), we worked with themes. After analysing the materials of each method separately, we grouped materials of different methods by theme. We tried to keep an open mind to avoid overlooking potential new themes.

4 Methodological Reflections

4.1 Drawing

In our study, making drawings proved to be a successful method. Most children liked it and completed the assignment in time. They were able to display what they considered important on their school route. Their drawings are mainly based on landmarks, which are among the destinations in the *third places* category. These landmarks are important points of reference that can help them find their way. According to Jansen-Osmann and Fuchs (2006), children are during wayfinding equally dependent on the existence of landmarks as adults. Children have a very good memory for landmarks, but are unable to locate them. This can also be seen in the drawings.

The drawings also reflect the meaning (part of the *Secondspace*) that children attribute to a place, since they represent the most important things on their route. This confirms

Cele's (2006) suggestion that drawings are influenced by previous experiences and context.

The majority of the children drew their school route as a single line or street with next to it buildings etc. drawn sideways (Fig. 1(Top)). This may suggest that the children were inspired by the teacher's example. Although the example was merely shown (as suggested by the teacher) to give an idea, while it was also mentioned that anything is allowed, many children seem to have followed it. We would advise other researchers not to give an example such that the children can fully use their imagination.

Older children are said to make more use of bird's eye view in their drawings (Cele 2006). In our study, some children rather used a combination of perspectives (Fig. 1 (Bottom)). This could indicate that they are already further in their development, have more imagination since they do not follow the teacher's example, or want to do something contrary by not following it.

4.2 Interviewing

During the interviews, the children enthusiastically talked about their own drawings. Conducting the interviews in groups of three, as recommended by Cele (2006), turned out to have advantages and disadvantages. In some groups there was interaction, but in others the children talked one by one and it did not really come to a discussion. This seems to confirm that keeping children's attention in the long term is more difficult (Rasmussen and Smidt 2003; Cele 2006). While we did follow the advice to use photos or drawings as a reference point, it was still difficult for some children to stay attentive.

4.3 Walking

The routes were determined during the preparation of the walks, but the children were allowed to lead the researchers. The routes also included 'unimportant places', such as *transitory zones*, which would not come up in a sedentary interview. During the walk, the researchers did not feel like they were in charge. This is not necessarily a disadvantage, since the children could walk around freely and react more spontaneously to space.

We divided the children in two groups to take two different walks. The children were given the role to guide the researchers. During the first walk, this role did not seem so clear to everyone. Moreover, asking interview questions during the walk not that easy – because the group was too large or children were busy exploring the area. The first walk took longer than expected: 1.5 h for a distance that would normally take 30 min to walk. This was actually positive: the second walk had to be postponed, offering us the opportunity to adjust our approach. Asking the questions no longer per stop for the entire group, but in a more spontaneous way during the walk, had a motivating effect on the conversations with the children. Perhaps they felt less crowded in smaller groups? The guides were also instructed in advance to look for places they (dis)liked. In this way their role was more clearly defined and they took it more seriously. The children told what they encountered along the way (e.g., 'this is a church', 'this is our old school') and took the lead. The places they mentioned were always landmarks, confirming their role in children's wayfinding.

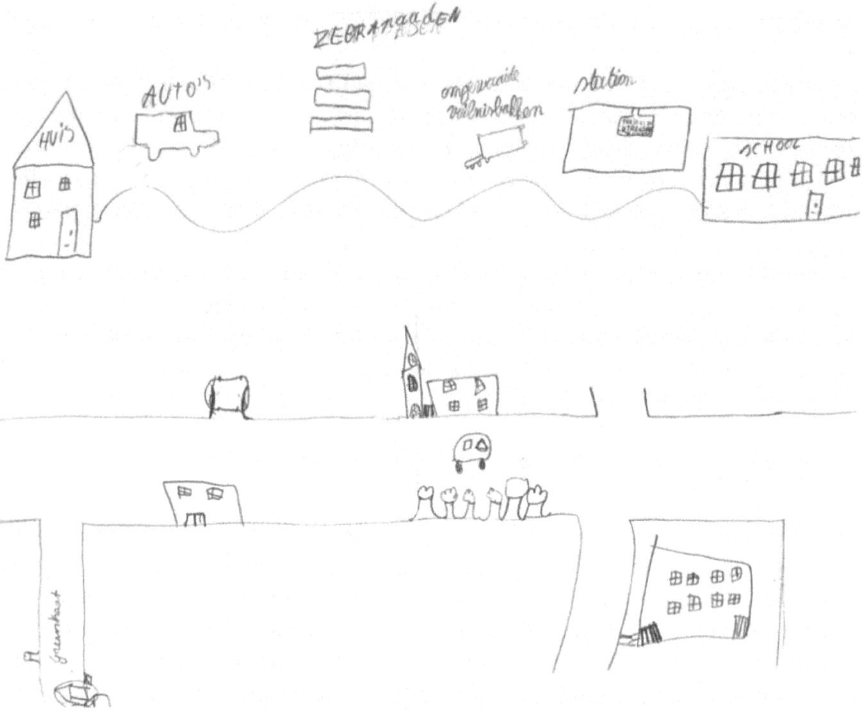

Fig. 1. Top: school route drawn as a single line/street and landmarks drawn sideways next to it. Bottom: school route combining bird's eye view (for the streets) and side view (for the buildings)

4.4 Photography

Using photography got the children to participate actively, enjoy the process, and be proud of their resulting photos. During the feedback moment, the children also received a printout of the photos, an important positive aspect of this method.

The photos indeed gave an indication of what children consider important. By taking photos, the children could express the meanings they attribute to their place experiences. Sometimes they even expressed an opinion within the photo itself by including their judgment (e.g., thumbs up for bicycles, thumbs down for cars). Many things they photographed are also reflected in the interviews and drawings. For example, they photographed each other while playing in places they know are intended for play (playgrounds, parks). These are mostly *destinations*, part of the *third places* (Oldenburg 1989). In other places, they did not photograph each other, although also there they started playing spontaneously. This sort of playing was mostly located in *transitory zones*.

Allowing children to show their perspective through photos offers insight into their place experiences. Partly due to their lower eye level, they are more attentive to things that often remain unnoticed for adults (Fig. 2).

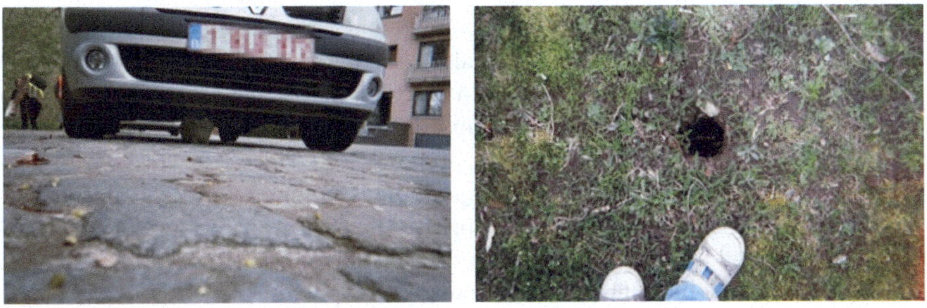

Fig. 2. Children have a lower point of view and are more attentive to things that often go unnoticed. Left: cat underneath a car; right: 'animal' hole

4.5 Feedback

During the feedback moment with the class, the first author presented all themes to the children, using their photos and drawings as reference points to ensure their interest. This allowed fine-tuning our findings with the help of the children. No new themes were identified, but for each theme extra information was added. The feedback moment showed that our interpretations of the children's drawings, interviews, walks, photos and conversations were mostly in line with their intentions. The discussion was useful to clarify a few things. For example, some photos turned out to be taken for a different reason than we had thought (e.g., a kitchen exhaust pipe was photographed because it looked 'cool', not because it was thought to be polluting the environment). A disadvantage of the class discussion was that often the same children spoke. The researcher tried to amend this by occasionally asking questions to children who were more quiet.

5 Discussion and Conclusion

Combining different methods in our study resulted in a considerable amount of material of different types (visual, auditive). This led to much information that was the same across methods, allowing to triangulate our findings. However, it also led to new themes that only came up in one source. In order to verify these new themes, it was important to discuss our interpretation with the children.

Using the conceptual framework was very helpful to structure and analyse the rich information we gathered, by looking in a more structured way at the materials. We have to keep in mind, though, that using other concepts could yield different findings.

The fact that we had time to improve our method for the walks, was positive. The first walk may seem less productive in terms of what we wanted to achieve, but when you 'invite the messy in research with children' (Elden 2013), it may be unavoidable to (keep) adjust(ing) your approach. Doing research together with children is first and foremost a learning process. We also found that it is important to take time for the walks, so as to allow for spontaneous detours and stops.

Besides our approach, working together with these children also gave us the opportunity to adjust our own perspective and biases. We learned that these children like quiet space, although in our society children are typically associated with noise. Also, the children are very curious about their environment and very much aware of it. And for some of the children who participated, social interaction includes animals.

The feedback moment with the children revealed that we interpreted some things differently than they do. This shows the importance of discussing interpretations with them.

All these findings teach us that children see things in their own way. It is thus very important to work together with them and involve them in research (or policymaking) from start to end, and for participation processes to evolve from consultation to cooperation. Moreover, while these processes are mostly set up with an eye to future changes, our study shows that it is also important to study how children see and do things in its own right.

References

Bishop K, Corkery L (2017) Designing cities with children and young people. Routledge, New York

Carroll P, Calder-Dawe O, Witten K, Asiasiga L (2019) A prefigurative politics of play in public places. Space Cult 22(3):294–307

Carroll P, Witten K, Stewart C (2017) Children are citizens too. Built Environ 43(2):272–289

Cele S (2006) Communicating place. PhD thesis, Stockholm University, Stockholm, Sweden

Coemans S, Vandenabeele J, Hannes K (2018) Een sensorische onderzoeksmethodologie. Sociologos 39(1):23–47

Cook T, Hess E (2007) What the camera sees and from whose perspective. Childhood 14(1):29–45

Dedding CW, Jurrius K, Moonen X, Rutjes L (eds) (2013) Kinderen en jongeren actief in wetenschappelijk onderzoek. Lannoo Campus, Houten

Elden S (2013) Inviting the messy. Childhood 20(1):66–81

Gardner PJ (2011) Natural neighbourhood networks. J Aging Stud. 25(3):263–271

Gibson JJ (1979) The ecological approach to visual perception. Houghton Mifflin & Co, Boston

Greene S, Hogan D (eds) (2005) Researching children's experience. Sage, London

Hackett A, Seymour J, Procter L (eds) (2015) Children's spatialities: embodiment, emotion and agency. Palgrave Macmillan, New York

Jansen-Osmann P, Fuchs P (2006) Wayfinding behaviour and spatial knowledge of adults and children in a virtual environment. Exp Psychol 53(3):171–181

Knowles-Yanez K (2005) Children's participation in planning processes. J Plan Lit 20(1):3–14

Mitchell LM (2006) Child-centered? Vis Anthropol Rev 22(1):60–73

Oldenburg R (1989) The great good place: cafes, coffee shops, bookstores, bars, hair salons, and other hangouts at the heart of a community. Paragon House, New York

Procter L, Hatton A (2015) Producing visual research with children: exploring power and meaning making. In: Stirling E, Yamada-Rice D (eds) Visual methods with children and young people. Academic and visual industries in dialogue. Palgrave Macmillan, Basingstoke

Raittila R (2012) With children in their lived place. Int J Early Years Educ 20(3):270–279

Rasmussen K, Smidt S (2003) Children in the neighbourhood: the neighbourhood in the children. In: Christensen P, O'Brien M (eds) Children in the city: home, neighbourhood and community. Routledge Falmer, Taylor & Francis Group, London, New York

Soja EW (1996) Thirdspace: journeys to Los Angeles and other real-and-imagined places. Blackwell, Oxford

Withagen R, Caljouw SR (2017) Aldo van Eyck's playgrounds. Front Psychol 8:1130

Moving Inclusively Through Transport Buildings: A Cross-disciplinary Design Case Study

J. Harding(✉)

WSP, Member of Wolfson College, Cambridge, RIBA, Cambridge, UK
john.harding@wsp.com

Abstract. Inclusivity within society is a critical pillar of sustainability. However, integrating cross-disciplinary thinking, user-centred and inclusive design paradigms within the built environment sector is a challenge. To address this concern, this study links and draws new meaning from a series of articles within the context of busy urban train stations. Questions addressed are: (i) what new guidelines could address inclusivity in practice? (ii) what underpinning theory, universal (UD) or inclusive design (ID) will satisfy inclusivity in practice? (iii) how could user-centric 'service design' (SD) methods be transferred to the built environment? (iv) what practical ways could audit inclusivity in the early design stage? (v) what new tools could be used to address cross-disciplinary and holistic thinking? (vi) how could a 'designerly way of knowing' technique address 'wicked' problems in inclusivity? and, (vii) what does design mean in this context? The study transfers 'SD' methods to the built environment to produce new insights.

1 The Rationale for the Study

The Bruntland Commission developed the concept that sustainable development is supported by the three pillars of economic growth, environmental protection and social equity (WCED 1987). Moreover, scholars recognise accessible public buildings and urban areas are critical to delivering products and services to people (Clarkson and Coleman 2015). Furthermore, it is known that complex socio-material interactions (Bichard 2014) impact user experiences (Battarbee and Koskinen 2005) and their inclusivity (Clarkson and Coleman 2015). For example, busy urban railway stations have complex public circulation layouts and low levels of inclusivity (Harding 2011). While it is recognised there is a need to develop guidelines for inclusivity within the built environment sector (Ormerod 2005; Sugiyama and Ward Thompson 2007, cited in Clarkson and Coleman 2015: 243) it is less understood what critical design guidelines are necessary and how they could be developed in practice. Consequently, the primary rationale is to probe how, passenger experiences of inclusivity are affected by the circulation layouts in stations.

Universal, accessible, adaptable and disabled are all euphemisms for the term disability, and this imprecise language harms academic discourse and the development of inclusivity within built environment (Bringolf 2009). Furthermore, inclusivity is a core

P. Langdon et al. (Eds.): CWUAAT 2020, *Designing for Inclusion*, pp. 115–122, 2020.
https://doi.org/10.1007/978-3-030-43865-4_12

commitment of the New Urban Agenda of UN-Habitat (adopted in 2016) and universal design (UD) is their preferred way to create inclusion (UN 2006). However, scholars argue UD aims to afford access to a wide range of users, whereas inclusive design (ID) aims to afford access to everyone (Martens 2018). Moreover, UD and ID have different theoretical underpinnings (Imrie 2012). Crucially, it is unknown what design paradigm produces satisfactory solutions for inclusivity in practice (Harding 2019). Consequently, the secondary rationale for this study is to probe what design paradigm (UD or ID) will satisfy inclusivity in practice.

Service design (SD) applies a five step methodology (see Fig. 1) to focus appropriate processes upon satisfying user needs (Bhavnani and Sosa 2008). SD is appreciated by scholars who specialise in ID (Clarkson and Coleman 2015). While SD is also used to design products (IDEO 2015) it is not used to design buildings. Instead, buildings are designed according to the canonical Plan of Work (RIBA 2013) used for the past 50 years (Sinclair 2013). And has seven stages (0-Strategic Definition, 1-Preparation and Brief, 2-Concept Design, 3-Developed Design, 4-Technical Design, 5-Construction, 6-Handover and Close Out, and 7-In use). It is argued that the Plan of Work reflects 'first-generation' design methods common in engineering disciplines owing to its positivistic, systematic, rational and scientific underpinnings (Rittel 1973 cited in Cross 2007: 1) that seeks to optimise the design (Cross 1982). Consequently, the third rationale probes to satisfy inclusivity in practice by asking how the Plan of Work could be revised to integrate SD methods.

Access audits are required to ensure compliance with legislation and are completed once the building is occupied (Ormerod 2005). However once occupied, it is costly and disruptive to modify the design of a building. Consequently, the fourth rationale considers what is a practical method to audit designs for inclusivity at the early design stage that is scalable, ethical, uses existing and trusted quantitative tools without the need for significant training?

Cross-disciplinary working practices within the built environment industry have increased costs and decreased productivity owing to poor collaboration and integration (Latham 1994; Egan 1998) and increasing sophistication, institutionalisation, industrialisation and complexity (Haenlein and Patel 2017). Furthermore, use of different underpinning theory and analytical tools among different disciplines result in a lack of holistic evaluation for technology that could satisfy inclusivity (Harding 2018b). For example, lift engineers analyse vertical movement of pedestrians within stations (Al-Sharif and Al-Adem 2014). In contrast, pedestrian modellers analyse horizontal and escalator pedestrian movements (Network Rail 2015). Consequently, the fifth rationale considers what new methods could integrate holistic and cross-disciplinary thinking in the early design stage.

Inclusivity in stations is a 'wicked' problem (Harding 2018b), meaning it is unlikely that all the information required to design a solution will be available, at the right time (Rittel and Webber 1973 quoted in Cross 1982). Consequently, the sixth rationale considers how could a '*designerly way of knowing*' (Cross 1982) be used to produce a 'design solution' that satisfies wicked inclusivity problems in practice.

Finally, 'design' has at least twelve meanings. Design is, (i) an affordance '*what it provides or furnishes, either for good or for ill*' (Gibson 1979: 127), (ii) a way of knowing (Cross 1982), (iii) a way to address 'wicked problems' (Cross 1982), (iv) a guessing game (Lawson 2004), (v) a favourable outcome for the user (Battarbee and Koskinen 2005), (vi) a process that is as important as the 'artefact' (Brandt 2006 quoted in Andrews 2014: 201), (vii) an activity (Lawson and Dorst 2013), (viii) a participatory process (Heylighen and Bianchin 2013), (ix) a long exploratory journey without clear or defined outcomes (Richard MacCormac cited in Lawson and Dorst 2013: 11), (x) a participatory endeavour (Cassim and Dong 2015), (xi) a limit for designers owing to 'design fixation' (Crilly 2015), and (xii) a consultation process with users of a building (Van der Linden et al. 2016). Consequently, the seventh rationale asks, what is design?

2 Methodology

To investigate these questions, this new synthesis draws upon SD methods and assembles and reflects upon earlier articles to produce a single case study. Case study methods can provide the reader with a broad understanding of the topic by using multiple sources of information to explicate the wider context (Yin 1993) and are common in the business (Creswell 2003) and built environment industries (Flyvbjerg 2006). The research design draws upon SD's five research steps (Bhavnani and Sosa 2008) see Fig. 1. Step 1 develops primary observational research (Harding 2011; Harding 2013; Harding et al. 2016). Step 2 synthesises earlier observations and literature into a new critical literature review (Harding 2018b). Step 3 develops new ideas to investigate inclusivity (Harding 2013). Step 4 refines a new methodology (Harding 2018a), and Step 5 implements that methodology in a new rival case study (Harding 2019).

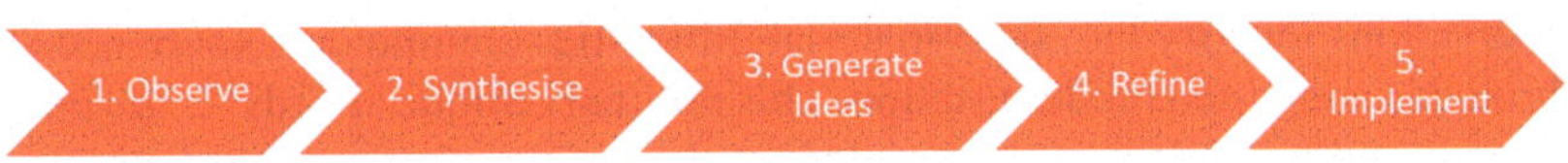

Fig. 1. Five service design steps (IDEO's model Bhavnani and Sosa 2008)

3 Summary of Results

Step 1 creates new observations within the context of busy urban railway station environments in London. Harding (2011) questionnaire survey explicates how gender and age affects a passenger's experience of inclusivity according to comfort, security, gentleness, and confidence experiences of 47 respondents (34 male, 13 female). Table 1 summarises differences in emoji and colour that indicate, (i) all groups had confidence, (ii) all groups had an ungentle experience, (iii) women, young and middle-aged groups require more comfort and security, and (iv) men require more comfort. Consequently, Table 1 provides a new "*... tool that compares experiences of different demographic groups, [to] promote reflexivity in practitioners who are working in uncertain, unstable, unique areas with conflicting requirements and values (Schon cited in Cross* 2007*: 3) and inform designers that other groups may have different experiences than their own (Warburton* 2003*; Marsden et al.* 2008*)*" (Harding 2018b).

Table 1. Comparing proxies for inclusivity to age and gender within busy train station contexts in London (modified from Harding 2011)

Proxies	Baseline	Young <25	Middle	Aging >55	Women	Men
Comfort	😐	☹	☹	☺	😐	😐
Security	☺	☹	😐	☺	😐	☺
Gentleness	☹	☹	☹	☹	☹	☹
Confidence	☺	☺	☺	☺	☺	☺
Satisfactory Experience= ☺ Middling Experience = 😐 Unsatisfactory = ☹						

A second observation study reports on critical socio-material interactions within the highly-acclaimed Canary Wharf underground train station building which opened in London in 2000 (Harding et al. 2016). The motivation for the study was to leave the design office and to observe how users interact with products (Battarbee and Koskinen 2005). It transfers auto-ethnographic qualitative methods of inquiry from social sciences to study socio-material interactions in underground train stations. To analyse the video files it revises an older method used to analyse audio files (Crichton and Childs 2005). New observations identify the socio-material difficulties commuters experience as they move through a congested modern station. This original critique affords "*... an insightful reflexive approach to begin to understand 'from the inside' why transport buildings pose particular challenges for inclusive design*" (Harding et al. 2016: 333).

Step 2 synthesises those step 1 observation studies with literature and develops a new cross-disciplinary body of literature that focusses upon the socio-material context of inclusive transport building design (Harding 2018b). Step 3 develops new ideas to reduce the impact of moving vertically and horizontally in crowded and busy stations (Harding 2013). Step 4 refines a new methodology to compare how rival designs impact inclusivity using agent-based modelling (ABM) (Harding 2018a). Step 5 implements the study and compares two rival design cases, see Fig. 2 (Harding 2019). Case 1 reflects UD and social model underpinnings (Vehmas 2008; Imrie 2012) and affords lift access for less than 10% of agents that does not provide access for a wide group of people (Martens 2018). In contrast, case 2 reflects ID and socio-material underpinnings (Slack 1999) and affords lift access for at least 25% of agents during the busiest peak period. In summary, the study revises design theory including, (a) highway and pedestrian movement theory (Fruin 1971) that uses Level of Service (LOS) to measure congestion can also be a valid new proxy to assess inclusivity in crowded buildings, (b) it is possible to increase LOS (or inclusivity) fivefold (case 2) by altering horizontal and vertical circulation including using multiple lifts, like a modern airport, without increasing the cost or size of the station.

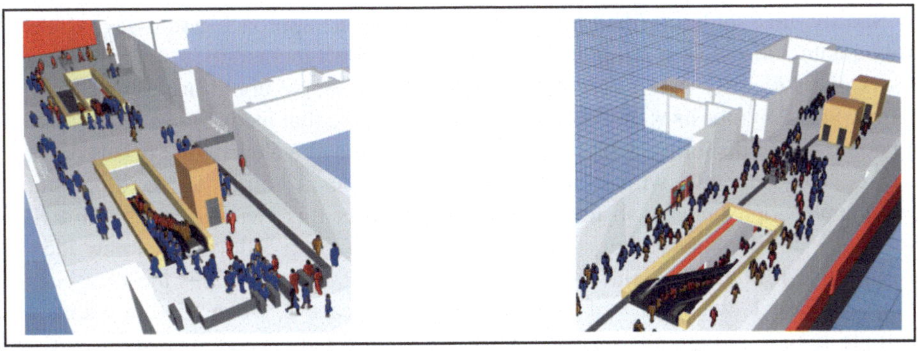

Fig. 2. Using agent-based-modelling to evaluate case 1 (left) and case 2 (right) for inclusivity

4 Conclusions and Innovations

Firstly, this study clarifies how adopting SD methods produces new design guidelines and layouts within the context of an ABM study for the first time. For example, step 1's observations identify a high level of crowdedness within poorly located and sized circulation elements as critical concerns for inclusivity. Step 2's synthesis identifies that only deep or **less busy** airport and terminus stations were considered suitable for multiple lifts (Fruin 1992). Step 3's new ideas aim to improve horizontal and vertical movement in the context of busy shallow urban underground stations. Step 4 refines that new idea by using a new ABM methodology to evaluate inclusivity. Step 5 implements that methodology to analyse inclusivity afforded by rival circulation arrangements.

Secondly, this study clarifies what design paradigm (UD or ID) will satisfy inclusivity in practice. Case 1 reflects how UD principles result in poor levels of access. On the other hand, case 2 reflects ID principles and contributes to the growing evidence that ID is the critical design paradigm that satisfies inclusivity (Martens 2018). Consequently, older views that UD creates inclusion (UN 2006) require revision.

Thirdly, while case 1 follows normal Plan of Work design stage, case 2 integrates the five SD (IDEO 2015) stages during the early stages of the Plan of Work'. While case 1 was unable to satisfy inclusivity, case 2 was shown to satisfy inclusivity in practice. In conclusion, SD can be considered a new 'next, next' generation design method '*more relevant to architecture and planning*' (Rittel 1973 cited in Cross 2007: 1).

Fourthly, this study clarifies how a new quantitative agent-based simulation methodology using LOS (Harding 2018a) was used in practice to audit the horizontal and vertical circulation systems at the early design stage. LOS is suggested as a new proxy to measure inclusivity. This innovation is scalable, ethical, and uses trusted quantitative tools that do not require significant training.

Fifthly, this study clarifies what cross-disciplinary working practices need integration to focus attention upon the user. These include, (i) integrating all vertical and horizontal movements in one model (see Fig. 2), (ii) revising older views that discount the use of lifts for moving large numbers of people (Network Rail 2015), (iii) revising theory that separates vertical movement via lifts (Al-Sharif and Al-Adem 2014) and pedestrian movement via escalators and passageways (Crooks et al. 2008).

Sixthly, this study clarifies how a design 'solution' approach addresses 'wicked' problems to address how many people require help with inclusivity at stations. Step 1 observations identify that a very small proportion of people could use a lift at a busy station. Step 2 synthesises this observation and literature that identifies as much as 20% of people have a disability, while many more people may be elderly, use prams or carry luggage. Consequently, with so many possible variables it is impossible to determine how many people may wish to use a lift. To address this 'wicked' problem a rival case study develops a 'design solution' (Cross 1982). Step 3 develops a new idea to use multiple lifts and straightforward access in case 2. Step 4 refines the idea. Step 5 compares case 1, when 10% of 'agents' use lifts, to case 2, when 25% of agents use multiple lifts. Consequently case 2 affords a five-fold increase in inclusivity with no additional cost or increase in size of the station. In conclusion, ABM as a tool and LOS as a proxy for inclusivity are suggested as valid new techniques to build trust in design solutions that address wicked and unknowable design and research problems. And, to satisfy inclusivity, it was possible to integrate SD's user-centric five step processes to evaluate and modify spatial arrangements in practice.

Finally, the meaning of design is sophisticated and contested. In conclusion, a discursive meaning for design is necessary to focus attention upon the complex, cross-disciplinary needs of the user. 'Next, next' generation 'SD' methods addressed complex 'wicked' problems. Consequently, this study reframes design as **a form of discourse.** This reframing may attract more researchers to use this approach owing to research is often considered a discourse. And, it is hoped that this study will inspire designers, researchers and policymakers to consider applying SD methods, not just in the design of services and products, but also to the design of the built environment so that everyone can "*...live and work in an inclusive world*" (Clarkson and Coleman 2015).

References

Al-Sharif L, Al-Adem MD (2014) The current practice of lift traffic design using calculation and simulation. Build Serv Res Technol 35:438–445

Andrews C (2014) Accessible participatory design: engaging and including visually impaired participants. In: Langdon PM et al (eds) Inclusive designing – joining usability, accessibility and inclusion. Springer, London

Battarbee K, Koskinen I (2005) Co-experience: user experience as interaction. CoDesign 1:5–18

Bhavnani R, Sosa M (2008) IDEO: service design. Insead, Paris

Bichard J-A (2014) Extending architectural affordance: the case of the publicly accessible toilet. PhD thesis, The Bartlett School of Architecture, University College London, London, UK

Bringolf J (2009) Calling a spade a shovel: universal, accessible, adaptable, disabled – aren't they all the same? In: Proceedings of the 4th Australasian housing researchers' conference, Sydney, Australia, 5–7 August 2009

Cassim J, Dong H (2015) Interdisciplinary engagement with inclusive design – the challenge workshops model. Appl Ergon 46:292–296

Clarkson J, Coleman R (2015) History of inclusive design in the UK. Appl Ergon 46(Part B):235–247

Creswell JW (2003) Research design: qualitative, quantitative and mixed methods approaches. Sage Publications, Thousand Oaks

Crichton S, Childs E (2005) Clipping and coding audio files: a research method to enable participant voice. Int J Qual Methods 4:1–9

Crilly N (2015) Fixation and creativity in concept development: the attitudes and practices of expert designers. Des Stud 38:54–91

Crooks A, Castle C, Batty M (2008) Key challenges in agent-based modelling for geo-spatial simulation. Comput Environ Urban Syst 32:417–430

Cross N (1982) Designerly ways of knowing. Des Stud 3:221–227

Cross N (2007) Forty years of design research. Des Stud 28:1–4

Egan J (1998) Rethinking construction, construction task force report for Department of the Environment, Transport and the Regions. HMSO, London, UK

Flyvbjerg B (2006) Five misunderstandings about case-study research. Qual Inq 12:219–245

Fruin JJ (1971) Pedestrian planning and design. Metropolitan Association of Urban Designers and Environmental Planners, New York, NY, US

Fruin JJ (1992) Designing for pedestrians. Public Transportation United States, Washington DC, US

Gibson JJ (1979) The theory of affordances. In: Gibson JJ (ed) The ecological approach to visual perception. Houghton Miffin, Hopewell

Haenlein H, Patel H (2017) Design-led procurement: linking the design process with procurement of construction projects. In: Hay R, Samuel F (eds) Professional practices in the built environment, conference proceedings, University of Reading, Reading

Harding J (2011) Investigating the built environment: Survey of inclusive design attitudes within London's tube stations. Departments of Engineering and Architecture, University of Cambridge, Cambridge, UK

Harding J (2013) Experiencing mobility in underground transport systems. In: Proceedings of LTA-UITP Singapore international transport congress and exhibition (SITCE 2013) LTA, Singapore, 7–10 October 2013

Harding J (2018a) Agent-based modelling could remove an ethical barrier to researching inclusivity in crowded places. In: Proceedings of the 9th Cambridge workshop on universal access and assistive technology, Fitzwilliam College, University of Cambridge, UK, 9–11 April 2018

Harding J (2018b) Fifty years of inclusive transport building design research. In: Roggema R et al. (eds) Proceedings of the 6th CIB international conference on smart and sustainable built environments, University of Technology, Sydney, Australia, 5–7 December 2018

Harding J (2019) Using agent-based modelling to probe inclusive transport building design in practice. Proc Inst Civ Eng – Urban Des Plan 172(3):111–123

Harding J, Luck R, Dalton NS (2016) Journeys in the city: empathising with the users of transport buildings. In: Proceedings of the international conference on integrated design. Building our future, University of Bath, Bath, UK, 30 June–1 July 2016

Heylighen A, Bianchin M (2013) How does inclusive design relate to good design? Designing as a deliberative enterprise. Des Stud 34:93–110

IDEO (2015) The field guide to human-centered design. IDEO org., Canada

Imrie R (2012) Universalism, universal design and equitable access to the built environment. Disabil Rehabil 34:873–882

Latham M (1994) Constructing the team. Final report of the joint government/industry review of procurement and contractual arrangements in the United Kingdom construction industry. HMSO, London, UK

Lawson B (2004) What designers know. Architectural Press, Oxford

Lawson B, Dorst K (2013) Design expertise. Architectural Press, Routledge, Abingdon

Marsden G, Cattan M, Jopson A, Woodward J (2008) Older people and transport: Integrating transport planning tools and user needs. Sparc, UK

Martens K (2018) Ageing, impairments and travel: priority setting for an inclusive transport system. Transp Policy 63:122–130

Rail Network (2015) Station capacity planning guidance. Network Rail, UK
Ormerod M (2005) Undertaking access audits and appraisals: an inclusive design approach. J Build Appraisal 1:140–152
Sinclair D (ed) (2013) RIBA plan of work 2013. RIBA, London, UK
Slack S (1999) I am more than my wheels. In: Corker M, French S (eds) Disability discourse. McGraw-Hill Education, Buckingham
UN (2006) Convention on the Rights of Persons with Disabilities and Optional Protocol. United Nations, New York, NY, US
Van der Linden V, Dong H, Heylighen A (2016) Capturing architects' designerly ways of knowing about users: exploring an ethnographic research approach. Design Research Society, Brighton, UK
Vehmas S (2008) Philosophy and science: the axis of evil in disability studies. J Med Ethics 34:21–23
Warburton N (2003) Everyday inclusive design. In: Clarkson J et al (eds) Inclusive design: design for the whole population. Springer, New York
WCED (1987) Our common future. Report of the World Commission on Environment and Development. Oxford University Press, UK
Yin RK (1993) Applications of case study research. Sage, London

Data and Inclusion: User Profiling

Ageing and Physical Activity: A Preliminary Literature Review

L. Liu[1,2] and H. Dong[2(✉)]

[1] College of Engineering, Nanjing Agricultural University, Nanjing, China
[2] School of Design and Creative Arts, Loughborough University, Loughborough, UK
{L.Liu2,H.Dong}@lboro.ac.uk

Abstract. Ageing is a prominent challenge facing the world. Increasing physical activity among older adults not only helps maintain and improve their health, but also has positive economic and social implications. Since 2007, research on physical activity among older adults has increased significantly, suggesting an increased research interest in the field. This paper reviewed relevant publication (from Web of Science Core Collection and Medline) over the period 1999–2019. The visualisation software CiteSpace was used to mine data, map information, and reveal trends. Important areas for further research were identified.

1 Introduction

Physical activity (PA) is an influencing factor for healthy ageing (Frank et al. 2012); the lack of PA has been associated with chronic diseases (Ashe et al. 2009; Marques et al. 2017). PA is a convenient, economical and effective means to cope with population ageing, and a 'miracle cure' to prevent and help treat many illnesses (CMO 2019). However, older adults are among the least physically active of all age groups (Levinger et al. 2018). Studies have been carried out to identify appropriate exercise interventions for older adults (e.g., Jia et al. 2018; Siemonsma et al. 2018), with controlled trial of exercise on physical function (Huang et al. 2015; Oesen et al. 2015; Sipila et al. 2018). In order to make better use of existing research to inform older adults's behaviour change and to inform future research directions, we carried out a preliminary literature review on ageing and physical activity.

2 Methods

To ensure the representativeness and authoritativeness of selected literature, *Web of Science Core Collection*, *Medline database* were selected as the source data. *Web of Science Core Collection* contains more than 12,000 authoritative and influential academic journals, while *Medline* is not only the largest database in *PubMed* system, but also the literature source of *Cochrane Library*, an authoritative database of evidence-based medicine. The combination of the two databases provides the literature for this review study. Using a Boolean search strategy, keywords were entered relating to the physical activity of older adults e.g., "physical exercise", "physical activity", "sports", "exercise facilities", "gym" and "older people", "elderly", "ageing". The time ranges from 1999 to 2019 (until September).

P. Langdon et al. (Eds.): CWUAAT 2020, *Designing for Inclusion*, pp. 125–131, 2020.
https://doi.org/10.1007/978-3-030-43865-4_13

2.1 Selection Criteria

First, the system filter of "Document Types" was used to focus on journal papers for better quality control. Then, the identified papers were reviewed by two independent researchers and the following criteria were used for exclusion:

- Duplication from the same author/similar research objectives or methods;
- No access to full texts (only abstracts available);
- Papers that are of a literature review nature;
- Content having less relevance to physical activity of older adults;
- Subjects under 60 years of age.

2.2 Data Visualisation

CiteSpace is the software for cluster analysis and visualisation, and it can help reveal research patterns and trends. In this study, CiteSpace.5.5.R2. was used to compile and analyse the data resulting from the review.

3 Results and Findings

The electronic search returned a total of 2448 papers (*Web of Science Core Collection*: 2196; *Medline*: 252). After using the system filter "Document Types", 2374 journal papers were retained. Using the exclusion criteria, 1405 papers were removed (duplication 187; no access to full text 113; other 1105) leaving 969 papers (*Web of Science Core Collection*: 878; *Medline*: 91) for review and analysis. Figure 1 shows the spread of papers over the period 1999-2019, suggesting a significant increase of numbers since 2007. One possible reason is the intervention of sports policies in various countries due to the declining or stagnant sport participation around the year of 2000 (Vail 2007), which aroused the interest of researchers. For example, the 'county sport partnerships' (CSPs) came into effect in 2003 in the UK and were extended to a larger national network of 49 partnerships with a much closer working relationship with National Governing Bodies (NGBs) in 2005 (Collins and Kay 2014). Canada issued the 'Physical Activity and Sport Act physical activity' in 2003 and the 'Integrated Pan-Canadian Healthy Living Strategy strategy' in 2005 (Wu and Zhang 2009). In 2006, the Chinese government issued the 'Eleventh Five-year Plan for Sports' and provided a series of policy support for the 2008 Olympic Games.

Figure 1 also reveals a pattern of a sudden increase of publications every three to four years since 2007, i.e., 2007, 2011, 2014, 2017. The general research period of two to three years may account for this phenomenon. The number of papers in 2019 is incomplete as the survey period ends in September 2019. The next significant increase may appear in 2020.

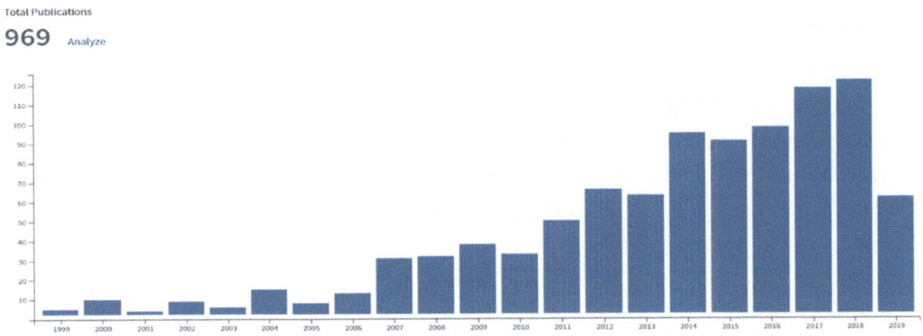

Fig. 1. Number of publications 1999–2019

3.1 Main Sources of Publication

The top seven sources of the publications are shown in Fig. 2. They are mainly medical journals, i.e., Medicine and Science in Sports and Exercise, Journal of the American Geriatrics Society, Archives of Physical Medicine and Rehabilitation, Jama-Journal of the American Medical Association, and American Journal of Preventive Medicine. Different from the young people who participate in physical activity mainly for the purpose of strengthening or shaping their body, most of older adults participate in physical activity for preventing chronic diseases or alleviating the symptoms of diseases to improve their quality of life (Luan et al. 2019). Exercise therapy research can provide guidance to family physicians and health management consultants to help develop personalised exercise prescriptions. This may explain why most publications are from medical journals rather than other fields.

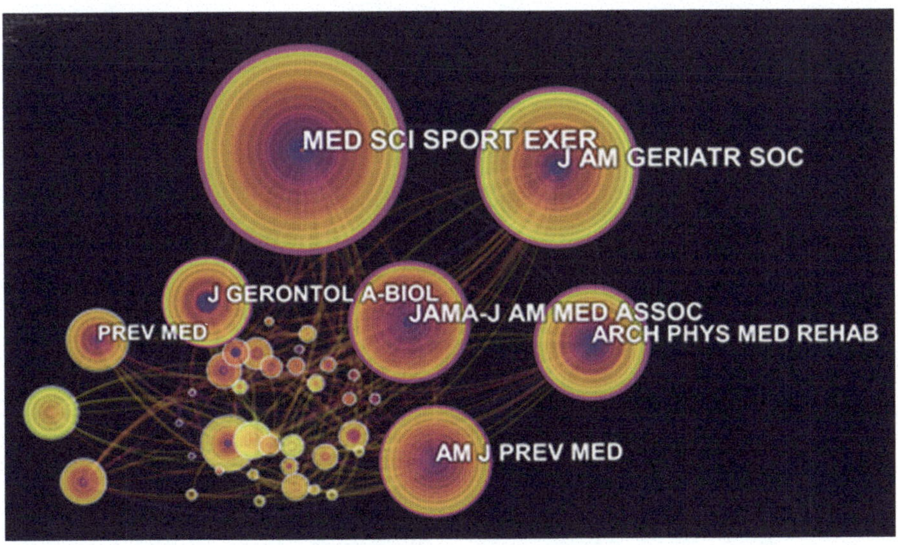

Fig. 2. Main sources of the publication

3.2 Fields and Keywords

Figure 3 illustrates a map of fields (in capital letters) and keywords (in lower case). Each node represents a different keyword, and the circles represent fields. The larger the 'cross' shape around a keyword (e.g., 'exercise'), the higher the frequency of the keyword. The larger the circles (e.g., 'REHABILITATION'), the more publication from the field.

4 Discussion

Based on the preliminary literature review, four insights have been gained:

Emerging Interdisciplinary Fields are Promising for Future Research. Existing research is mainly focused on the medical field, and some new trends of interdisciplinary research have emerged, for example 'nursing home characteristics' (Akihiro et al. 2018; Yang et al. 2019). Physical activity is an individual behaviour that is influenced by interpersonal (Markland and Tobin 2010), environmental (Pyky et al. 2019) and policy factors (Troped et al. 2001). Therefore, the study of physical activity for older adults should involve a wider range of disciplines.

Further Development of Theories are Needed. Although some research results show that taking regular physical activity can improve older adults' cognitive function (Pereira et al. 2019), regulate their psychological mood and maintain a good state of mind (Leung et al. 2004), theories are still lacking: e.g., the mechanism of the effect of physical exercise on cognitive ability of older adults, the 'dose-effect' relationship between physical activity and cognitive function.

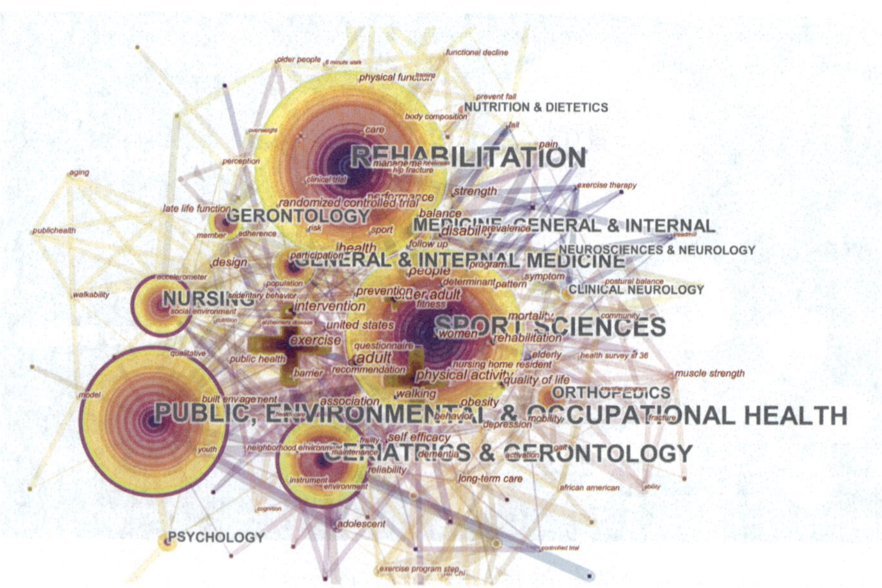

Fig. 3. Fields and keywords mapping

Outdoor Exercise Needs More Attention. There is emerging evidence of significant psychological and cognitive benefits accruing from regular exercise participation by older adults (Chodzko-Zajko et al. 2009). A study has shown promising effects on self-reported mental wellbeing immediately following exercises in nature which is not seen following the same exercise indoors (Coon et al. 2011). However, few older people exercise outdoors other than walking. How to effectively promote outdoor exercise among older adults? What policy and interventions are needed? What outdoor facilities are required? And how to ensure safety and easy access? These all need further research.

The Impact of Design on the Uptake of Physical Activity Needs Investigation. Most publications from medical fields involve exercise intervention, controlled trials, empirical analysis, and policy-making and programming. Fitness equipment, exercise facilities and products also affect older adults' participation of physical activity, in addition to the factors such as environment (Calogiuri and Elliott 2017), accessibility (Calder et al. 2018) and operation (Hunter et al. 2015) discussed in the existing literature. Therefore it is worth investigating whether design factors also affect older adults' participation in physical activity.

Moreover, we have identified three areas for future research:

- To explore the mechanism of physical and psychological effects of physical activity on older adults, with a focus on developing theoretical frameworks;
- To utilise knowledge and expertise from sports, sociology, psychology, medicine and design in future research; to study the mechanism of the effect of physical exercise on cognitive ability of older adults;
- From the perspective of user experience, to study how outdoor exercise facilities affect older adults' participation in physical activity and improve the ease of use and satisfaction with outdoor exercise provision.

References

Akihiro S, Taira Y, Maeda K, Natsume K, Sakakima H (2018) Feasibility and effectiveness of home-based exercise programs on physical performance and health-related quality of life of the older people dwelling on an isolated doctor-less island. Geriatr Gerontol Int 18(9):1313–1317

Ashe MC, Miller WC, Eng JJ, Noreau L (2009) Older adults, chronic disease and leisure-time physical activity. Gerontology 55(1):64–72

Calder A, Sole G, Mulligan H (2018) The accessibility of fitness centers for people with disabilities: a systematic review. Disabil Health J 11(4):525–536

Calogiuri G, Elliott LR (2017) Why do people exercise in natural environments? Norwegian adults' motives for nature-, gym-, and sports-based exercise. Int J Environ Res Public Health 14:377

Chien KY, Chang WG, Sanders ME, Chen CH, Wu WC et al (2019) Effects of land vs water jump exercise: implications for exercise design targeting bone health. Scand J Med Sci Sports 29(6):826–834

Chodzko-Zajko WJ, Proctor DN, Fiatarone MA, Minson CT, Nigg CR et al (2009) Exercise and physical activity for older adults. Med Sci Sports Exerc 7:1510–1530

Collins M, Kay T (2014) Sport and social exclusion, 2nd edn. Routledge, Abingdon

Coon JT, Boddy K, Stein K, Whear R, Barton J et al (2011) Does participating in physical activity in outdoor natural environments have a greater effect on physical and mental wellbeing than physical activity indoors? A systematic review. J Epidemiol Community Health 65:1761–1772

Frank W, Christian K, Matthew J (2012) Lack of exercise is a major cause of chronic diseases. Compr Physiol 2(2):1143–1211

Hita-Contreras F, Bueno-Notivol J, Martinez-Amat A, Cruz-Diaz D, Hernandez AV et al (2018) Effect of exercise alone or combined with dietary supplements on anthropometric and physical performance measures in community-dwelling elderly people with sarcopenic obesity: a meta-analysis of randomized controlled trials. Maturitas 116:24–35

Huang TT, Liu CB, Tsai YH, Chin YF, Wong CH (2015) Physical fitness exercise versus cognitive behavior therapy on reducing the depressive symptoms among community-dwelling elderly adults: a randomized controlled trial. Int J Nurs Stud 52(10):1542–1552

Hunter RF, Christian H, Veitch J, Astell-Burt T, Hipp JA et al (2015) The impact of interventions to promote physical activity in urban green space: a systematic review and recommendations for future research. Soc Sci Med 124:246–256

Jia XJ, Yu Y, Xia WN, Masri S, Sami M et al (2018) Cardiovascular diseases in middle aged and older adults in China: the joint effects and mediation of different types of physical exercise and neighborhood greenness and walkability. Environ Res 167:175–183

Leung KK, Wu EC, Lue BH, Tang LY (2004) The use of focus groups in evaluating quality of life components among elderly Chinese people. Qual Life Res 13(1):179–190

Levinger P, Sales M, Polman R, Haines T (2018) Outdoor physical activity for older people – the senior exercise park: current research, challenges and future directions. Health Promot J Austr 29(3):1036–1073

Luan X, Tian XY, Zhang HX, Huang R, Li N et al (2019) Exercise as a prescription for patients with various diseases. J Sport Health Sci. 8(5):422–441

Markland D, Tobin VJ (2010) Need support and behavioural regulations for exercise among exercise referral scheme clients: the mediating role of psychological need satisfaction. Psychol Sport Exerc 11(2):91–99

Marques A, Peralta M, Martins J, de Matos MG, Brownson RC (2017) Cross-sectional and prospective relationship between physical activity and chronic diseases in European older adults. Int J Public Health 62(4):495–502

Oesen S, Halper B, Hofmann M, Jandrasits W, Franzke B et al (2015) Effects of elastic band resistance training and nutritional supplementation on physical performance of institutionalised elderly – a randomized controlled trial. Exp Gerontol 72:99–108

Oh S-L, Kim HJ, Woo S, Cho BL, Song M et al (2017) Effects of an integrated health education and elastic band resistance training program on physical function and muscle strength in community – dwelling elderly women: healthy aging and happy aging II study. Geriatr Gerontol Int 17(5):825–833

Pereira T, Rao S, Pandey A, Garg S, Park B et al (2019) Exercise, ageing and cognitive function – effects of a personalized physical exercise program in the cognitive function of older adults. Physiol Behav 202:8–13

Pyky R, Neuvonen M, Kangas K, Ojala A, Lanki T et al (2019) Individual and environmental factors associated with green exercise in urban and suburban areas. Health Place 55:20–28

Siemonsma PC, Blom JW, Hofstetter H, van Hespen ATH, Gussekloo J et al (2018) The effectiveness of functional task exercise and physical therapy as prevention of functional decline in community dwelling older people with complex health problems. BMC Geriatr 18(1):164

Sipila S, Tirkkonen A, Hanninen T, Laukkanen P, Alen M et al (2018) Promoting safe walking among older people: the effects of a physical and cognitive training intervention vs. physical training alone on mobility and falls among older community-dwelling men and women (the PASSWORD study): design and methods of a randomized controlled trial. BMC Geriatr 18(1):215

Troped PJ, Saunders RP, Pate R, Reininger B, Ureda JR et al (2001) Associations between self-reported and objective physical environmental factors and use of a community rail-trail. Prev Med 32(2):191–200

Vail SE (2007) Community development and sport participation. J Sport Manage 21(4):571–596

Wu YH, Zhang WW (2009) The study on sports legislation of Canada. J Hubei Sports Sci 28(3):274–276

Yang LJ, Wu GH, Yang YL, Yang LJ, Wu GH et al (2019) Nutrition, physical exercise, and the prevalence of sarcopenia in elderly residents in nursing homes in China. Med Sci Monit 25:4390–4399

Detail Matters: Exploring Sensory Preferences in Housing Design for Autistic People

P. Nguyen[1,2](✉), V. d'Auria[3], and A. Heylighen[1]

[1] Department of Architecture, Research[x]Design, KU Leuven, Leuven, Belgium
{phuong.nguyenlan,ann.heylighen}@kuleuven.be
[2] Faculty of Architecture and Planning, National University of Civil Engineering, Hanoi, Vietnam
phuongnl@nuce.edu.vn
[3] Department of Architecture, OSA, KU Leuven, Leuven, Belgium
viviana.dauria@kuleuven.be

Abstract. Autistic people deal with their environment in a unique way due to differences in sensory perception. Designing housing for autistic people who are unknown is challenging. This research aims to help bridge the gap between architects' design intentions and autistic users' experiences. By combining interviews and participant observation, a case study of a residential facility shows how autistic users can experience things differently than architects assume. Differences relate especially to noise and temperature perception, the size of shared rooms, and visual stimulation in private units. Sensory preferences incorporated in the design based on particular examples of sensory symptoms within the autism spectrum do not necessarily match the preferences of the actual users. This case study contributes to an accumulative knowledge base of thoroughly studied housing designs for autistic people.

1 Introduction

Sensory perceptual differences represent a major aspect of autism[1] (American Psychiatric Association 2013). Examples include hyper- or hypo-sensitivity to sensory stimuli, inability to filter sensory information, fragmentation of information, or delayed processing (Bogdashina 2016). Because of these differences in sensory perception, autistic people[2] deal with their environment in a unique way, which affects how they experience and interact with the surrounding world (Kinnaer et al. 2016). Often they live in environments that do not take into account their responses to sensory input (Brand and Gaudion 2012).

Sensory accessibility is a major theme in the literature on designing for autism (Kinnaer et al. 2016). Sensory preferences are incorporated in architectural design as

[1] Autism refers to a range of conditions related to social behaviour, communication and language, and a narrow range of interests and activities that are unique to the individual and carried out repetitively (World Health Organization 2018).

[2] The term 'autistic people' tends to be preferred by autistic adults, whereas professionals rather prefer 'person with autism' (Kenny et al. 2016).

P. Langdon et al. (Eds.): CWUAAT 2020, *Designing for Inclusion*, pp. 132–139, 2020.
https://doi.org/10.1007/978-3-030-43865-4_14

a sensory design approach for autism (Mostafa 2008). This approach tends to balance sensory experiences (Kim and Sherry 2015), e.g., by creating a sensory neutral residence where visual, acoustic, olfactory and tactile qualities can be easily modulated to suit a resident's particular preferences (Brand 2010), or by creating different rooms so that residents can choose the suitable sensory environment for themselves (Mostafa 2008; Brand 2010).

The sensory design approach shows limitations. Concepts used can be interpreted in multiple ways (Kinnaer et al. 2016). For example, whereas one autistic person prefers open spaces because the overview they offer makes things predictable, another autistic person prefers compartments, as they reduce sensory input and offer structure (Kinnaer et al. 2014). Researchers developed design guidelines (Kim and Sherry 2015; Gaines et al. 2016), based on experimental (Mostafa 2008; Brand 2010; Khare 2010) and feedback studies (Whitehurst 2007; Scott 2009), yet these focus mostly on hypersensitivity (Kim and Sherry 2015) – possibly because some researchers oversimplified sensory perceptual differences within the autism spectrum (Bogdashina 2016). Additionally, evidence-based studies about designing for autistic users are still limited.

When designing accommodation for autistic adults living independently, architects may adopt the sensory design approach to adjust their design to autistic users' needs. To help bridge the gap between architects' intentions and users' experiences, our case study seeks to answer the following questions: (1) how are sensory preferences within the autism spectrum incorporated in architects' design intentions? And (2) how do autistic residents experience the resulting environment? In addressing these questions, we hope to enrich the understanding of sensory preferences in the context of housing design for autistic people - among architects, developers and care professionals who may reconsider their position and seek opportunities to improve autistic people's quality of life.

2 Methods and Materials

In order to gain an in-depth understanding of architects' design intentions and autistic residents' experiences, we adopted a qualitative research approach that combines interviews and participant observation. The first author – henceforth 'the researcher' – has a background in architecture and residential planning. She developed skills in communicating and interacting with autistic people, within the context of the Relationship Development Intervention programme (Gutstein and Sheely 2002) and her own family. The second and third authors have backgrounds in architecture, design research and anthropology.

The selected case is Peacefield,[3] a residential facility designed to provide independent living conditions supervised by coaches[4] for 20 autistic residents with mild mental retardation or an average IQ. It is located in a quiet area in the middle of a residential block, in a low-density residential district at the outskirts of a city. Situated in the middle

[3] To omit details that might allow participants' identification, the setting's and participants' names were pseudonymised. However, the illustrations may enable people familiar with the setting to recognise it.

[4] A coach is a professional care provider, Flemish word is 'woonbegeleider', meaning guide or counsellor.

of the site, the building consists of staggered volumes, intended to emphasise dwelling rather than institutional care. Individual residential units are articulated by alternating roof heights, like the pitched roofs of many Belgian town-houses, and town-house windows (Fig. 1a, b).

Based on the ratio of 1 coach to 5 residents, each dwelling module is called a 'house'. The five private units are spread along a curved corridor, at the end of which there is a shared living room with a working desk for the coach. There are two houses on the ground floor and another two on the first floor. Two modules on the same floor are connected through a corridor and share a bathroom, time-out and laundry rooms (Fig. 1c). Each resident rents a private unit as a fully equipped, small apartment. It has an entrance, cabinet and shower room. Depending on the resident's preference, there is a kitchen, and a removable wall allows the unit to be a bedroom with a separate living room (Fig. 1d) or a large studio (Fig. 1e).

The person in charge of Peacefield's infrastructure – henceforth the developer – was interviewed informally (for two hours). From the team of five architects who designed the project, semi-structured interviews were conducted jointly with two architects – Peter and Leon – and separately with the interior architect – Maria (for 90 min each). Participating residents were chosen based on the researcher's informal contacts during participant observation, and in consultation with coaches. Coaches were chosen based on their availability. Eight residents – Charles, Anthony, Barbara, Emily, Antoine, Mitch, Dan and Fischer – and four coaches – Ellen, Kelly, Neville and Lea – were informally interviewed about their experiences. Participants had been living or working in Peacefield for about two to four years. Residents (2 women, 6 men) were between 19 and 63 years old, coaches (3 women, 1 man) between 30 and 50. They were free to choose the language in which to communicate with the researcher. Most of them preferred English, except

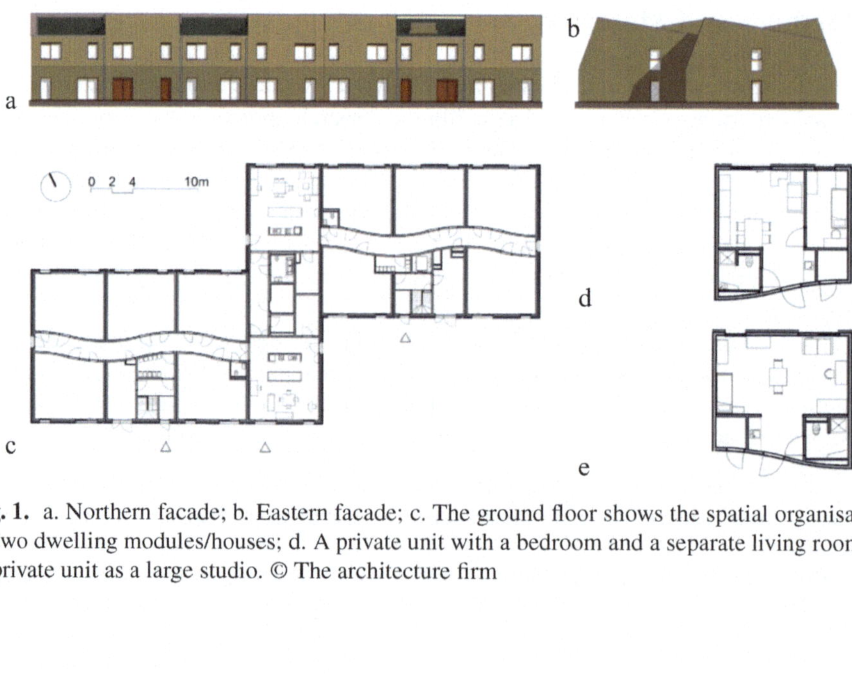

Fig. 1. a. Northern facade; b. Eastern facade; c. The ground floor shows the spatial organisation of two dwelling modules/houses; d. A private unit with a bedroom and a separate living room; e. A private unit as a large studio. © The architecture firm

for one resident who preferred French, and another for whom an assistant translated between Flemish and English.

Data collected include notes, pictures, drawings from residents, drawings provided by architects, the design brief from the developer, and audio recordings.

The developer was asked to recount her knowledge about autistic people and Peacefield's ambition, and to describe the building and how it was for residents to live there; the architects were asked to recount their acquaintance with autistic people and their design intentions during the design process.

In Peacefield, 55 h of participant observation focused on daily activities of residents and coaches at different times within one month (June 2018). The researcher's participation included talking to residents and coaches, cooking, joining residents during dinners, working in the Peacefield and communal garden, going out (for walks, to the spa by car, or out dancing). The researcher took notes on a laptop at the table in the shared living room, similar to how coaches did administrative tasks. The observations allowed the researcher to become acquainted with residents and coaches, the built environment, and daily activities. This helped to better understand and interpret interview data within their context.

Combining participant observation with interviews allowed to explore residents' experiences. In the interviews, residents were asked, first, to guide the researcher through their private units and, second, to describe their private unit to the best of their ability, how it was for them to live in their private unit and in Peacefield, and what they did or would like to do. Of the 8 residents, 4 made drawings about their private unit, the building and residential area. This made it easier to communicate their thoughts, allowing more time to reflect and think while offering an opportunity to avoid eye-contact. In follow-up interviews they talked about their drawings, which helped in understanding their experiences.

Finally, coaches were asked to describe the building, their role in the house, how it was for residents to live there, and what they consider essential for residents.

Data analysis focused on interviews with all participants, complemented by observation notes, drawings, pictures, and the design brief. It roughly followed QUAGOL (Dierckx de Casterlé et al. 2012) and used qualitative data analysis software (Nvivo 11). To gain thoughtful insight into the data (Dierckx de Casterlé et al. 2012), the analysis was conducted in consultation and through discussion with the second and third author. The third author also read transcripts and made narrative reports.

The study was approved by KU Leuven's ethical committee. Participants were informed about the study orally and in written form, and given the opportunity to ask questions. The interviews with residents were adapted to their individual capacities in terms of timing, length, and content. All interviewed residents said to feel comfortable doing the interview alone and gave written informed consent.

3 Findings

3.1 Sensory Preferences in Architects' Design Intentions

The architects highlighted themes like 'individualisation', 'homeliness' and 'sensory preferences'. Incorporating the latter appeared to be a primary design strategy and profoundly influenced decisions throughout the design process.

The architects seemed to be aware of the differences in sensory perception within the autism spectrum. During the design process, Maria and Leon spent a day and talked with the staff at another residential setting for autistic people managed by the same developer. Several severe sensory symptoms were considered during the design. Examples include someone who could count into hundreds if he saw 100 tiles, could hear a tapping pen from another room, could not sleep because of noise from the ventilation, or unscrewed his bed after one night. Sensory preferences from these accounts were used to question everything during the design process.

> *"Not everyone is sensitive with hearing or not everyone is fixed on a screw, depending on who will be living there, you can adjust and give more freedom or less freedom … I have (a) few faces in my head, so, when William is in there what we will do? It made it just easier to control your design somewhat and it made especially with colours and materials, it made a lot of decisions."*
>
> (Interview Maria)

Architects' design intentions incorporated several sensory preferences. The primary design strategy was to create a low-stimulation environment by minimising visual stimuli in several ways: introducing a curved corridor to avoid hard edges (as these might create unpredictable confrontation between residents) (Figs. 1c and 2); minimising window details by installing a window fitting to be flush with the wall; using large-size (90 × 90 cm) bathroom tiles for walls and seamless, continuous floors and ceilings (incorporating lights) to reduce the number of joints; using neutral colours, and underfloor heating in order to avoid radiators.

Particular attention was paid also to acoustic solutions: situating the building centrally on the site created a buffering area which reduces noise from the surroundings; double walls between units and sand-lime brick absorb sounds, a green roof absorbs noise from rain, and an extra layer buffers sound from the roof; sloped walls and roof should reduce the sound reflection on the first floor; ventilation shafts run separately to the basement to avoid sound travelling between units; and underfloor heating avoids sounds from running water inside radiators.

Finally, the architects intended to offer individual units more space than shared rooms – unlike in the older group living facility managed by the developer, where individual units have limited space and shared rooms are much bigger.

3.2 Autistic Users' Experiences

In autistic residents' experiences, themes that stood out include 'autonomy' and 'sensory preference'.

A major concern for users is noise inside the building: the robust material in the corridor causes echo to occur (Fig. 2); a small detail of the lock used on all doors creates a loud sound each time a door is (un)locked; residents tend to check the lock multiple times; and the solution for sound absorption between floors is insufficient. A battle between residents was reported because of noise caused by a first floor unit.

> *"Some inhabitants have very highly sensitive hearing, so, if, they are also afraid of the door. If one of the doors closes, some [...] inhabitants here can hear it. They are very nervous, very angry. It is, almost, noise cannot escape."*
>
> (Interview Fischer)

According to the coaches, a second major concern for the residents is the temperature. Since residents cannot control it by themselves, it relates to the theme of autonomy.

> *"The feeling of warm, cold, and they cannot adjust it by themselves. It is a problem... it's hard to explain to the technician to arrange the temperature, because they say 'No, it's 21 degree, it's fine like that'. But NO, we have COLD, and we have to use trousers. Because the feeling is not, eh, like that."*
>
> (Interview Ellen)

3.3 Confronting Design Intentions with User Experiences

A commonality between the architects' design intentions and users' experiences concerns the size of the private units. Most participating residents appreciated their spacious private unit where they could "escape" from outside sensory stimulation, relax, do their stuff. Charles named it his "escape room".

Differences concern the noise inside the building and the room temperature. Other differences were observed in relation to the size of the shared room and the visual stimulation in private units. While the architects intended to reduce the shared living rooms in size, some residents occupy more space than others according to their sensory preferences. For example, Mitch preferred to lean on the kitchen counter and observe

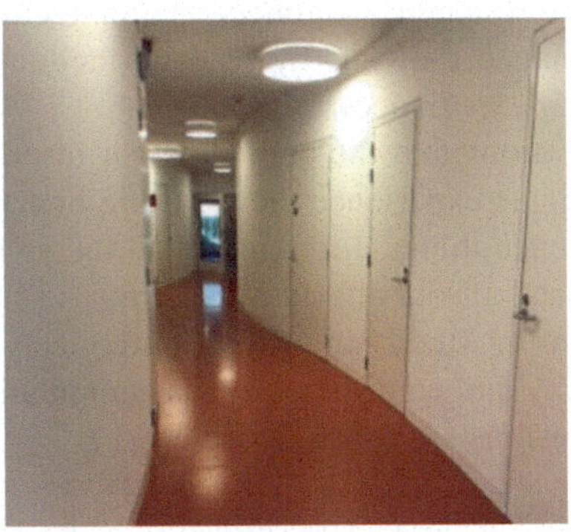

Fig. 2. 'Noisy' corridor with robust material

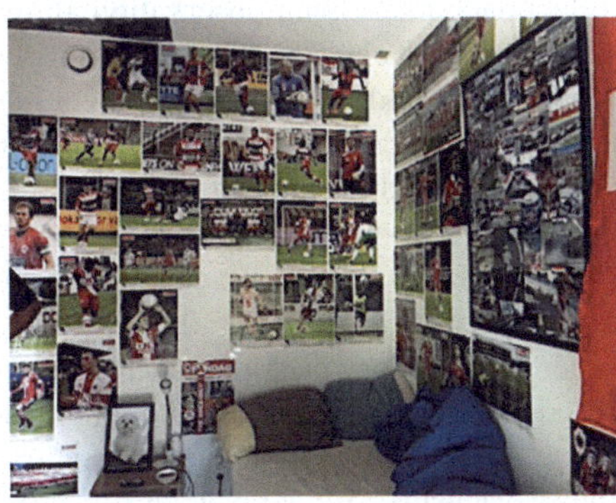

Fig. 3. Walls full of posters in Antoine's private unit

people from a distance rather than using the sofa. Barbara was keeping a distance from others, using her straight arm to measure her private space. She did not sit with others at the shared dining table, her table was set apart. Some residents occupied more space by moving their body to regulate their emotions and sensory inputs. For example, Barbara walked back and forth, rocked her body when she was nervously searching cheese for her diner sandwiches. Fischer walked back and forth when he was excited having his new game device on hands. The coaches admitted that the shared rooms were too small. Inside 5 private units, there were varieties of visual stimuli with many little things which relates to their personal interest, e.g., displayed collections of cigars, newspapers, CD-ROMs, posters, Pokémon images, decorating lights, Pop game figures or other stuff (Fig. 3). Unlike the architects' intention to minimise visual stimulation, those displays, presented to the researcher during the guided visit of the private units, were visibly essential in the residents' units.

4 Discussion and Conclusion

Incorporating sensory preferences profoundly shaped architects' intentions from the conceptual to the interior design stage. The users' experiences actually differed from what the architects had assumed, especially related to noise and temperature; the size of the shared room; and visual stimulation in the private units. More space is needed in the shared room to allow some autistic people to regulate emotions and/or sensory inputs. This is in line with Scott's (2009) finding that classrooms for autistic children require more space than those for neurotypical children. Minimising visual stimulation would be more important in the shared rooms than in private units. Some autistic people need visual stimuli, which might relate to sensory fascination (Bogdashina 2016).

Sensory preferences from particular (extreme) examples within the autism spectrum do not necessarily match the sensory preferences of the actual users. As Bogdashina (2016) claims, autistic people often describe their stims as defensive mechanisms. Attention should focus on civilising the sensory environment rather than judging autistic people's behaviour (Davidson and Henderson 2016).

In terms of limitations of the study, the language used for interviews was neither the participants' nor the researcher's mother tongue. Yet, additional techniques were used to collect data: participant observation allowed the researcher to reflect on architectural aspects of the built environment and users' performance; drawings by residents facilitated communication and offered more insight into their experiences.

The study offers insight into the design intentions that the architects put in practice and a nuanced account of how autistic residents experience the resulting housing environment. Autistic users turned out to experience things differently than the architects assumed. Detail matters: despite the architects' all-out efforts, something as small as a lock became a big issue. The insights from the study may support architects in incorporating sensory preferences in a tailored way and contributes to an accumulative knowledge base of thoroughly studied housing designs for autistic people.

Acknowledgements. We are grateful to the developer, architects, coaches and residents who generously gave of their time and energy for this study. This research was supported by Vietnam International Education Development.

References

American Psychiatric Association (2013) DSM5 diagnostic criteria autism spectrum disorder. In: Diagnostic and statistical manual of mental disorders, 5th edn. American Psychiatric Association, Arlington

Bogdashina O (2016) Sensory perceptual issues in autism and Asperger syndrome: different sensory experiences – different perceptual worlds, 2nd edn. Jessica Kingsley Publishers, London

Brand A (2010) Living in the community housing design for adults with autism. www.rca.ac.uk/documents/390/Living_in_the_Community.pdf. Accessed 13 Dec 2019

Brand A, Gaudion K (2012) Exploring sensory preferences – living environments for adults with autism. Helen Hamlyn Centre for Design Royal College of Art, London

Davidson J, Henderson VL (2016) The sensory city: autism, design and care. In: Bates C et al (eds) Care and design: bodies, buildings, cities. Wiley, Chichester

Dierckx de Casterlé B, Gastmans C, Bryon E, Denier Y (2012) QUAGOL: a guide for qualitative data analysis. Int J Nurs Stud 49(3):360–371

Gaines K, Bourne A, Pearson M, Kleibrink M (2016) Designing for autism spectrum disorders, 1st edn. Routledge, New York

Gutstein S, Sheely RK (2002) Relationship development intervention with children, adolescents and adults: social and emotional development activities for Asperger syndrome, autism, PDD and NLD. Jessica Kingsley Publishers, London

Kenny L, Hattersley C, Molins B, Buckley C, Povey C et al (2016) Which terms should be used to describe autism? Perspectives from the UK autism community. Autism 20(4):442–462

Khare R (2010) Designing inclusive educational spaces for autism. Institute for Human Centered Design, Boston

Kim S, Sherry A (2015) At home with autism: designing housing for the spectrum. Policy Press, Bristol

Kinnaer M, Baumers S, Heylighen A (2014) How do people with autism (like to) live? In: Langdon PM et al (eds) Inclusive designing: joining usability, accessibility and inclusion. Springer, Cham

Kinnaer M, Baumers S, Heylighen A (2016) Autism-friendly architecture from the outside in and the inside out: an explorative study based on autobiographies of autistic people. J Housing Built Environ 31(2):179–195

Mostafa M (2008) An architecture for autism: concepts of design intervention for the autistic user. J Archit Res 2(1):23

Scott I (2009) Designing learning spaces for children on the autism spectrum. BILD Br Inst Learn Disabil 10(1):36–51

Whitehurst T (2007) Evaluation of features specific to an ASD designed living accommodation. Technical report, Sunfield Research Institute, Stourbridge

World Health Organization (2018). Autism spectrum disorders, 2 April 2018. www.who.int/news-room/fact-sheets/detail/autism-spectrum-disorders. Accessed 17 Aug 2019

Quantifying Exclusion for Digital Products and Interfaces

J. Goodman-Deane(✉), M. Bradley, S. Waller, and P. J. Clarkson

Cambridge Engineering Design Centre, University of Cambridge, Cambridge, UK
{jag76,mdb54,sdw32,pjc10}@cam.ac.uk

Abstract. It is useful to be able to estimate the numbers of people who are likely to be unable to complete task steps in a user journey and thus are excluded from using a product or service. This helps to identify and prioritise design issues and can lead to improvements in design. Existing approaches to quantifying exclusion have proven valuable for non-digital products and services. However, they do not explicitly take into account additional factors that impact digital interface use, such as technology experience and willingness to explore an interface. Digital inclusion is increasingly important as many services now incorporate digital interaction patterns. Thus it would be valuable to extend exclusion analysis into the field of digital interfaces. To this end, this paper proposes a new model of digital exclusion. The model is supported by the identification of key user characteristics that affect digital exclusion. We also outline three different approaches for using this model in practice to estimate the inclusivity of a digital interface.

1 Introduction

Digital inclusion is increasingly important as many services move online or incorporate digital interaction patterns. These include essential services, such as government information, banking and shopping. People who are unable to access and use digital technologies are increasingly likely to be excluded from many aspects of participation in society. Furthermore, they miss out on opportunities that could make life easier for them or enable them to stay independent for longer. This is a particular issue for older people, with adults over 65 having significantly lower rates of technology use (Office of National Statistics 2018). They are therefore likely to have less familiarity with digital interaction patterns.

There has been substantial interest in quantifying the numbers of people who are digitally excluded (e.g., OECD 2001; Cruz-Jesus et al. 2012). However, much of this work takes a broad standpoint, assuming that each person is either included or excluded. This is useful for policy making but less useful for improving individual services and interfaces. In reality, exclusion varies depending on the particular digital technology. Someone may be able and willing to use one piece of technology (e.g., a familiar e-mail client on a computer) but be completely confused by another (e.g., a navigation app on a smartphone). Another person may have access to the internet in their home but not on the move.

We propose addressing this by examining digital exclusion on the level of individual interfaces in specific target use settings. This could help designers to identify and

P. Langdon et al. (Eds.): CWUAAT 2020, *Designing for Inclusion*, pp. 140–149, 2020.
https://doi.org/10.1007/978-3-030-43865-4_15

prioritise exclusionary usability issues with their interfaces, help companies to choose between different possibilities, and assist in identifying gaps in provision from a broader perspective.

This is an approach that has been used successfully with non-digital products (Goodman-Deane et al. 2018a), as described in the following section. However, extending the approach to digital interfaces requires some modifications. In this paper, we describe how the underlying model of demand and exclusion can be adapted for digital interfaces, identify key user characteristics that affect digital exclusion, and outline three different approaches for using the model in practice to estimate the inclusivity of a digital interface.

2 Background

The exclusion estimation approach is based on the model of product interaction shown in Fig. 1 (Persad et al. 2007). Product interaction places demands on users' capabilities. Users will be excluded from using a product if any of its demands are higher than their capabilities.

Estimating exclusion uses this model by breaking down the use of a product into a series of tasks. The assessor evaluates each individual task against the points on various

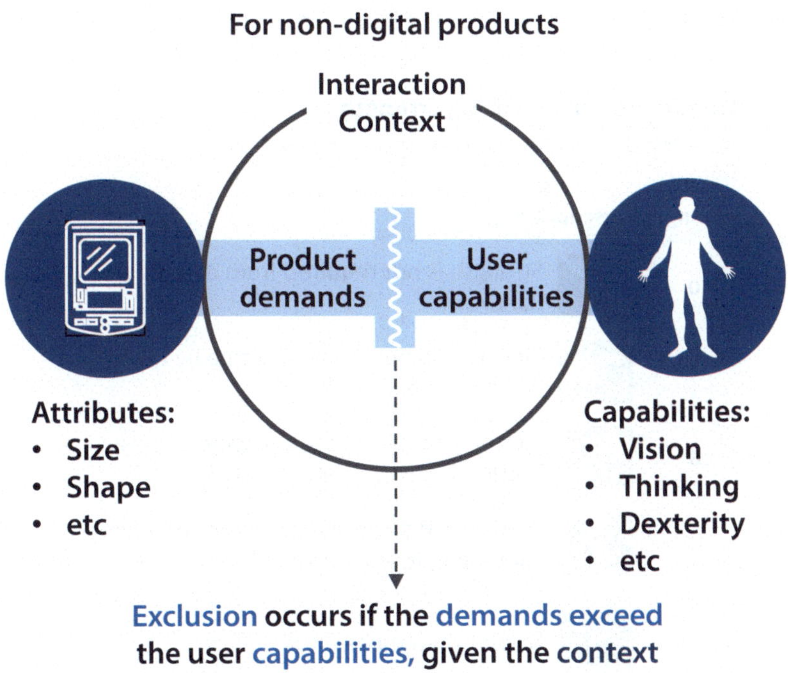

Fig. 1. Model of demand and exclusion for non-digital products (redrawn from Persad et al. 2007). Users will be excluded from using a product if any of its demands are higher than their capabilities

capability demand scales, such as vision and lifting strength (Fig. 2) (Waller et al. 2010). For example, a kettle that needs to be filled manually (and thus carried while full) requires a high amount of lifting strength. These demands are then compared with data on the spread of users' capabilities in the UK population, using Exclusion Calculator software (Cambridge Engineering Design Centre 2017). This estimates how many people would be unable to do that task in practice, e.g. how many people lack the strength capability to lift the full kettle.

It is important to note that operating most products requires a combination of several different capabilities, such as vision, dexterity and cognition. Thus, to estimate exclusion accurately, survey data is needed that covers multiple capabilities for each individual. To address this, the exclusion calculator uses data from the UK Disability Follow-up Survey (Grundy 1999) that covers motor, sensory and some cognitive capabilities.

It is recommended that exclusion calculations are complemented by other methods including user observation, user trials and expert appraisals to provide a more complete picture of the user interaction.

This approach has been insightful when used in collaboration with companies on non-digital products. The results from user trials are particularly effective in highlighting real issues, and the exclusion calculations help to indicate the prevalence of these issues in the wider population. This has helped to convince designers and managers of the need for more inclusive design, to break them out of a mindset of designing for people with similar capabilities to themselves or making guesses as to where users may struggle, and to educate them on what product attributes are likely to cause exclusion. It has

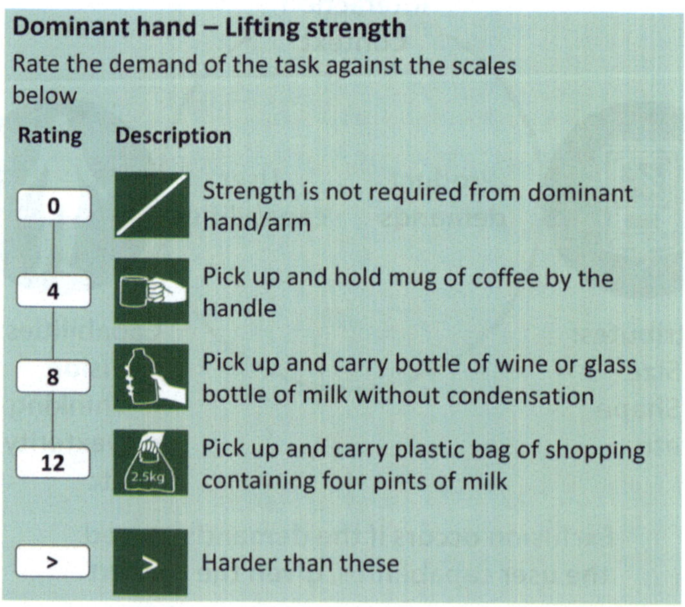

Fig. 2. One of the scales in the current exclusion calculator (Cambridge Engineering Design Centre 2017). Assessors compare the demand of the task against the points on the scale

identified areas that need to be improved, encouraged clients to make changes and enabled comparison of product alternatives (Goodman-Deane et al. 2018a).

3 A Model of Exclusion for Digital Interfaces

The model of exclusion shown in Fig. 1 is based on the theory that exclusion occurs if the demands of a product exceed the user's capabilities, given the context. This holds true for digital interfaces as well. For example, an interface may require the user to remember what they typed in on a previous screen. This places a sizeable demand on the user's memory capabilities.

However, this does not cover the whole picture. Successful use of a digital interface may depend on other aspects as well as the user's capabilities (see, e.g., Murad et al. 2012). For example, the interface may assume a user has knowledge of certain digital interaction patterns, a compatible learning style or attitude towards technology. It may be difficult for users to use the interface effectively if they do not have these characteristics. Many of these characteristics are not intrinsic human capabilities, and some cannot easily be conflated onto ordinal scales. As a result, it may not be possible to determine precisely whether a digital interaction demand exceeds a user's level of the characteristic.

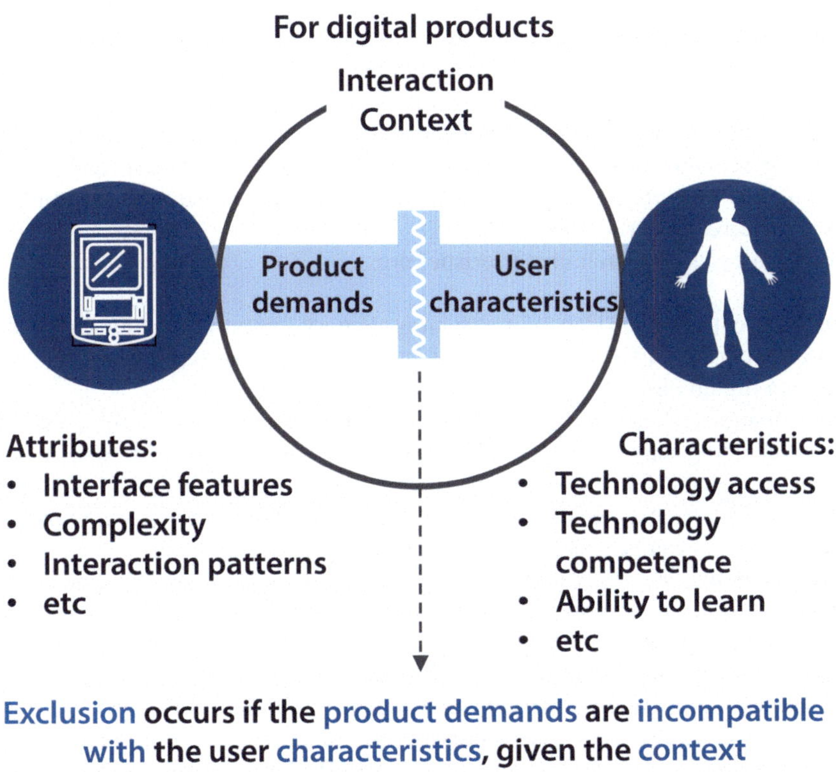

Fig. 3. Adaptation of the model of demand and exclusion from Fig. 1 for digital products

To address this, we propose modifying the model of exclusion as shown in Fig. 3. The user is now considered in terms of characteristics rather than capabilities, and exclusion now occurs if the product demands are incompatible with the user characteristics, given the context. A demand is considered to be incompatible with a user's characteristics if it requires something of the user (and their characteristics) that is not available in that context.

For some interface attributes, this is similar to the previous model. For example, a piece of text on a screen can cause exclusion because it is incompatible with the user's vision capability. It requires a level of vision from the user that they do not possess. This is the same as the vision demand exceeding the vision capability in the previous model.

However, for other attributes, it goes further. A service could be incompatible with a user's learning style and willingness to explore. The user may be unable to use the interface effectively in practice because they do not engage in the expected exploratory behaviours. In another example, it could be incompatible with a user's technology access because it demands a technology set-up that the user is not able to achieve given the technology available to them and their expertise in manipulating that technology.

4 User Characteristics Affecting Digital Exclusion

The new model (Fig. 3) considers each user in terms of their *user characteristics*. However, the term *characteristics* is extremely broad. It is possible to identify an enormous set of characteristics of users, many of which have little or no bearing on their use of technology, e.g., their hair colour or favourite food. It is important to narrow down the set and identify the key types of characteristics that affect the ability to use a digital interface. We conducted a literature review on this topic and identified several key areas, as shown in Fig. 4. Unfortunately, there is no room in this paper to describe the full range of papers referred to during this.

In summary, the key user characteristics are:

- **Cognitive capabilities:** Capabilities such as memory, executive function and attention play an important part in the use of digital interfaces, which are typically more complex than non-digital ones.
- **Neurodiversity:** Neurodiversity is a broad term, covering many neurological differences, including autism, ADHD and dyslexia. Many of these affect the ways in which people approach and interact with interfaces. Some interface attributes can be particularly difficult for people with certain characteristics. For example, text in particular fonts or colours can be problematic for some people with dyslexia.
- **Technology access:** Many interfaces require access to additional equipment and/or infrastructure to work properly. For example, a mobile data connection or a device with a certain specification may be required. It is important to note that technology access varies by situation as well as by person.
- **Technology competence:** Competence varies between interfaces, but there are key underlying skills that can be transferred to a new interface. Competence itself can be hard to measure quickly. However, it is heavily influenced by technology prior experience and it may be possible to estimate it in some cases using prior experience

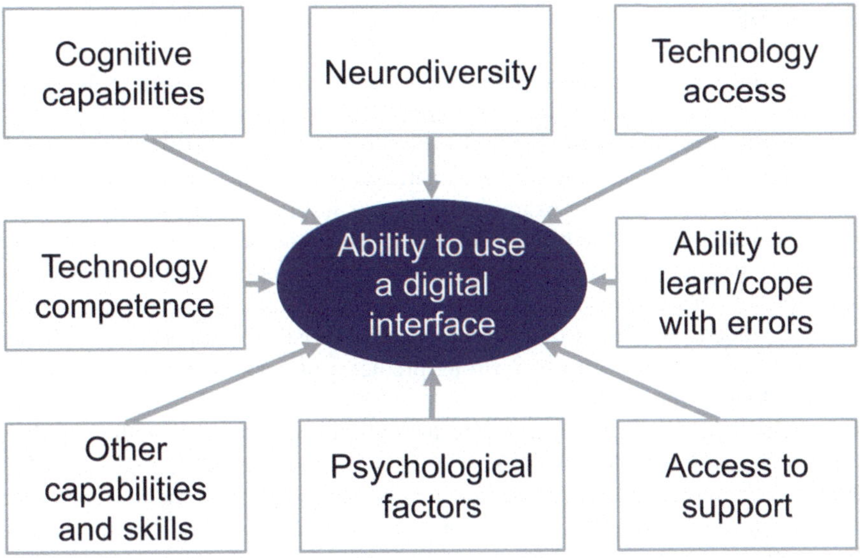

Fig. 4. Key user characteristics that affect a person's ability to use a digital interface. This was based on a literature review, with particular reference to Barnard et al. (2013) and Wagner et al. (2010)

(Blackler et al. 2010). It is also closely related to constructs such as intuitive use of technology (Blackler et al. 2010).

- **Ability to learn and cope with errors:** Digital interfaces often require users to learn new things. Even an interface that is similar to a familiar one will likely have some new aspects to learn, such as new sequences of button presses to achieve goals. Learning style can also be an issue. For example, many digital interfaces assume a level of willingness to explore or tinker with an interface and certain information processing styles, which vary across the population, e.g., by age and gender (Burnett et al. 2016). The ability to cope with and recover from errors is also critical in using digital interfaces. A well-designed interface with clear options for undoing actions can place less demand on this ability.
- **Other capabilities and skills:** These include sensory and motor capabilities, literacy and language.
- **Psychological factors:** Factors such as motivation, attitude to risk and technology self-efficacy (a person's beliefs about their ability to learn and use technology) can play a big part. For example, a complex-looking piece of technology may deter someone with low self-efficacy from trying it out, even if that person actually possesses the levels of capability required to operate it.
- **Access to support:** A person may be able to use an interface on a daily basis but will need help to set it up and if something goes wrong. If there is no one to provide support in these situations, they will be excluded from using the technology in practice. It is debatable if this is really a user characteristic or part of the interaction context. However, in either case, it affects digital exclusion.

5 Challenges

The method for estimating non-digital exclusion was outlined in Sect. 2. However, it may be difficult to use this in a digital setting for various reasons.

Firstly, there are a large number and variety of user characteristics that affect digital exclusion. In addition, some of these characteristics are hard to measure, and vary depending on the situation. For example, a person's level of confidence or self-efficacy may change depending on the particular interface they are facing. One possible way of addressing this is to consider subsets of characteristics that override or predict others. For example, if someone does not have the requisite technology access then they are probably excluded, regardless of their other characteristics. Furthermore, technology competence has been shown to be a strong predictor of performance on its own (e.g., Sengpiel and Dittberner 2008).

Other challenges arise when trying to match interface elements with user characteristics. It is possible to do this (at least roughly) with many aspects of a non-digital product. For example, an expert assessor may be able to give a rough estimate of the level of vision needed to read a piece of text (in a given context, e.g., without a screen reader or other assistive technology present). Doing this is also possible for some of the characteristics that affect digital exclusion, such as technology access. However, this is much more challenging when considering cognitive and expertise demands. For example, it is very difficult to determine the level of memory required to use an interface or a menu structure, or the level of expertise or prior knowledge needed to operate an unfamiliar app.

In addition, some of the characteristics that affect exclusion are not ordinal. Examples include learning style and aspects of neurodiversity. Such characteristics cannot be placed in a scale from low to high. As a result, it may not be possible to determine a particular "level" of the characteristic that is required to use an interface successfully.

Another issue is that different people use interfaces in different ways to achieve the same goals. One example of this is the use of assistive technology, such as a screen reader. Another example is the use of a wizard interface to achieve a goal that might be done more directly by someone with more experience. As a result, it may be necessary to examine multiple pathways in a task analysis and perhaps determine which one(s) are mostly likely for different people and situations.

6 Possible Approaches for Estimating Digital Exclusion

User trials are a key way to identify usability problems. However, it can be difficult to obtain a population-level view of exclusion with user trials without involving a large variety (and hence large number) of people. Therefore, in this section, we first focus on expert appraisal methods that utilize data about the spread of characteristics across the population as a whole. Section 6.3 then discusses how such data could be combined with user trials.

6.1 Compare Characteristics for Each Individual in a Dataset

The non-digital exclusion estimation method (described in Sect. 2) examines each person in a dataset in turn. For each individual, it compares their capabilities with the demands of the task to determine if they can do the task successfully.

Despite the challenges described in Sect. 5, it may be possible to use a similar method for digital interfaces, though it may be necessary to focus on just a few of the characteristics that impact digital exclusion. One possibility is the approach proposed by Bradley et al. (2018). In this approach, the assessors first perform a task analysis. For each task, they examine whether it requires the use of a digital interaction pattern. If it does, they determine whether the action required by the user is explicitly obvious for someone with no prior digital experience, e.g., if it maps "directly to an interaction pattern in the analogue world" (Bradley et al. 2018). If not, then the step is marked as exclusionary for everyone in the dataset with no prior experience of that particular interaction pattern (Bradley et al. 2015).

This method has the advantage that thousands of individuals in a dataset can be processed easily by a computer, comparing their known characteristics with the requirements of the tasks. However, it requires that a single task analysis be constructed that applies to all users, even though in practice different users approach an interface differently. It is possible to calculate exclusion for tasks that can be achieved in multiple different ways (Waller et al. 2013). However, the complexity of the task analysis, and the computation and interpretation of results increases dramatically as the number of different ways increases.

6.2 Quantitative Personas

A second possibility is to use quantitative personas as proposed in Goodman-Deane et al. (2018b). This method leverages personas that have been created from survey data using cluster analysis. Each persona is a fictional description of a user that represents a cluster or group of people in the population. They include information on the whole range of characteristics that impact digital exclusion. The assessor examines each persona in turn to determine if they would be able to complete the task with the digital interface. If they can, then it is assumed that the group they represent can do it too (and vice-versa).

This method allows an expert assessor to consider separately how each persona would approach a task. It also provides greater flexibility in considering how different user characteristics interact in particular situations. However, there is a trade-off between the number of personas that can feasibly be considered, and the validity of the assumption that "if a persona is excluded, then everyone in the cluster they represent would be excluded" (Goodman-Deane et al. 2018b).

6.3 Combining User Trials with a Dataset

Another approach, currently being developed by the authors, integrates user trials with survey data. In this approach, participants in user trials are given simplified versions of the survey questionnaire. The results enable the researchers to identify how many people in the survey (and thus in the wider population) are similar to each participant in terms of the characteristics that affect digital exclusion. The results from the user trials can therefore be quantified in population terms by assuming that if the participant in the user trial was excluded, then each person in the survey who is 'similar' to that participant will be excluded. Furthermore, the survey data can be examined to identify segments of the population who are not similar to any of the participants who have been recruited so far. This can be used to identify the extent to which the current user trial participants cover the diversity found in the wider population, and therefore to plan further recruitment.

This method is more expensive than the expert appraisal methods described earlier, but combines the advantages of both user trials and population figures.

7 Conclusions and Further Work

In this paper, we have presented a model of how digital exclusion arises due to mismatches between a product's demands and a user's characteristics. This is an adaptation of an earlier model that examined exclusion in non-digital products and services. We have also identified a wide variety of user characteristics that affect a user's ability to use a digital interface and thus whether they are digitally excluded.

This model can be used to estimate how many people in a population would be unable to achieve particular tasks with a digital interface (and would thus be digitally excluded). We have described some of the challenges in doing this and suggested some promising approaches to deal with these.

All of these methods rely on having good-quality survey data about how the user characteristics vary across the target population. Therefore, we have recently conducted a survey of 338 people aged 16+ across England and Wales. The survey covered technology access, experience and expertise, attitudes towards technology, sensory, physical and cognitive capabilities, and demographics. Initial results can be found in Goodman-Deane et al. (2020). We are currently analysing the results of this survey to be used with the various approaches outlined in Sect. 6. This will help to determine which approaches are most promising in practice. Further work will examine whether exclusion estimates based on this data correspond to actual performance on usability tests.

Acknowledgements. This work, funded by the Department for Transport (DfT), was delivered through RSSB's TOC'16 project: Towards the Inclusive Railway. Collaborative partners were Siemens Mobility, Keolis Amey Docklands and Astutim.

References

Barnard Y, Bradley M, Hodgson F, Lloyd A (2013) Learning to use new technologies by older adults: perceived difficulties, experimentation behaviour and usability. Comput Hum Behav 29(4):1715–1724

Blackler A, Popovic V, Mahar D (2010) Investigating users' intuitive interaction with complex artefacts. Appl Ergon 41:71–92

Bradley M, Kristensson PO, Langdon P, Clarkson PJ (2018) Interaction patterns: the key to unlocking digital exclusion assessment? In: Proceedings of AHFE 2018, Orlando, FL, US, 21–25 July 2018

Bradley M, Langdon P, Clarkson PJ (2015) Assessing the inclusivity of digital interfaces – a proposed method. In: Universal access in human-computer interaction. Access to today's technologies, Proceedings of UAHCI 2015, Los Angeles, CA, US, 2–7 August 2015

Burnett M, Stumpf S, Macbeth J, Makri S, Beckwith L et al (2016) GenderMag: a method for evaluating software's gender inclusiveness. Interact Comput 28(6):760–787

Cambridge Engineering Design Centre (2017) Exclusion calculator. http://www.calc.inclusivedesigntoolkit.com. Accessed 9 Sept 2019

Cruz-Jesus F, Oliveira T, Bacao F (2012) Digital divide across the European Union. Inf Manag 49:278–291

Goodman-Deane J, Bradley M, Clarkson PJ (2020) Digital technology competence and experience in the UK population: who can do what. In: Proceedings of ergonomics and human factors 2020, Stratford-upon-Avon, UK, 27–29 April 2020

Goodman-Deane J, Waller S, Bradley M, Bradley O, Clarkson PJ (2018a) Using inclusive design to drive user experience improvements through to implementation. In: Langdon PM et al (eds) Breaking down barriers: usability, accessibility and inclusive design. Springer, Switzerland

Goodman-Deane J, Waller S, Demin D, González-de-Heredia A, Bradley M et al (2018b) Evaluating inclusivity using quantitative personas. In: Proceedings of DRS 2018, University of Limerick, Limerick, Ireland, 25–28 June 2018

Grundy E (1999) Great Britain Department of Social Security Disability in Great Britain: Results from the 1996/97 disability follow-up to the family resources survey. DSS Report 94. Corporate Document Services, London, UK

Murad S, Bradley M, Kodagoda N, Barnard Y, Lloyd A (2012) Using task analysis to explore older novice participants' experiences with a handheld touchscreen device. In: Anderson M (ed) Contemporary ergonomics and human factors 2012. CRC Press, Boca Raton

OECD (2001) Understanding the digital device. OECD Publications, Paris

Office of National Statistics (2018) Internet access – Households and individuals, Great Britain. www.ons.gov.uk/peoplepopulationandcommunity/householdcharacteristics/homeinternetandsocialmediausage/bulletins/internetaccesshouseholdsandindividuals/2018. Accessed 9 Sept 2019

Persad U, Langdon P, Clarkson PJ (2007) Characterising user capabilities to support inclusive design evaluation. Univ Access Inf Soc 6(2):119–135

Sengpiel M, Dittberner D (2008) The computer literacy scale (CLS) for older adults – development and validation. In: Proceedings of Mensch und Computer 2008, Luebeck, Germany, 7–10 September 2008

Wagner N, Hassanein K, Head M (2010) Computer use by older adults: a multi-disciplinary review. Comput Hum Behav 26:870–882

Waller SD, Bradley MD, Langdon PM, Clarkson PJ (2013) Visualising the number of people who cannot perform tasks related to product interactions. Univ Access Inf Soc 12(3):263–278

Waller SD, Langdon PM, Clarkson PJ (2010) Using disability data to estimate design exclusion. Univ Access Inf Soc 9(3):195–207

Accessibility Barriers

Measuring the Time Impact of Web Accessibility Barriers on Blind Users: A Pilot Study

M. Griffith[1], B. Wentz[2](✉), and J. Lazar[3]

[1] Trace Center, HCIL, College of Information Studies, University of Maryland, College Park, MD, USA
meaggrif@umd.edu
[2] Shippensburg University, Shippensburg, PA, USA
bwentz@ship.edu
[3] Trace Center, HCIL, College of Information Studies, University of Maryland, College Park, MD, USA
jlazar@umd.edu

Abstract. As governments around the world increase or clarify the requirements related to web accessibility for public accommodations, they often require some level of cost-benefit analysis for the proposed regulation. As a part of these cost-benefit analyses, it's important to understand not only the costs of making technology accessible, but also the costs (in terms of the value of time) to Blind users (and people with other disabilities) of not making the technologies accessible. Furthermore, as the next generation of accessibility guidelines are in development, it's important to understand which specific accessibility barriers have the greatest impact on the productivity of users. This paper presents a literature review on the topic and also a discussion of two proposed methodologies for quantifying the impact of accessibility barriers by collecting time data on the difference between websites designed with high accessibility and those that have poor accessibility. Results from a pilot study of the first methodology will be presented.

1 Introduction

Numerous studies over the years have documented accessibility-related barriers in various categories of websites. Generally, these barriers impact Blind users the hardest, as the barriers tend to be most problematic for screen reader users. However, the studies often focus on determining the presence of accessibility barriers, rather than determining the specific impact of those barriers. What has not yet been quantified is the impact that these accessibility barriers have, in terms of the increased amount of time that it takes Blind users to accomplish tasks.

In the U.S., government agencies at the federal level are legally required to make their websites (and other technologies) accessible for people with disabilities, under Section 508 of the Rehabilitation Act. State and local government must make their websites accessible under Title II of the Americans with Disabilities Act (Lazar et al. 2015). Any private organization that is classified as one of the 12 categories of public accommodations under Title III of the Americans with Disabilities Act must also make its website accessible. On 15 January 2019, the U.S. 9th Circuit Court of Appeals reversed

P. Langdon et al. (Eds.): CWUAAT 2020, *Designing for Inclusion*, pp. 153–160, 2020.
https://doi.org/10.1007/978-3-030-43865-4_16

a lower court decision, reaffirming yet again that the Americans with Disabilities Act addresses websites of public accommodations, even in the absence of specific technical guidance or regulations on what interface accessibility standards to use (Lf legal 2019). Also, in October 2019, the U.S. Supreme Court refused to review the Robles v. Domino's Pizza case at that time (known as a "denial of a petition for a writ of certiorari") letting the 9th circuit's decision stand (Bloomberg 2019).

In the U.K., the Equality Act 2010 prohibits exclusion from the use of services because of a disability, and this includes online services (GEO 2015). Under this legislation, providers must make "reasonable adjustments" to the services that they offer online. To strengthen the Equality Act 2010, a new regulation was enacted called the Public Sector Bodies (Websites and Mobile Applications) (No. 2) Accessibility Regulations 2018. This new regulation requires new public sector websites and mobile applications to be accessible, but it also required existing public sector websites to be made accessible by September 2020 (2021 for mobile applications). This includes compliance with WCAG 2.1 AA and the publication of an accessibility statement (National Archives 2018). Since 2014 in the EU, the European standard for digital accessibility is a guideline known as EN 301 549 (EFTA 2014). The premise of this standard for the public sector is that all information and communication technology (including websites) needs to be accessible to everyone, which includes people with disabilities. Similar to the UK regulations, EN 301 549 has been updated to point to WCAG 2.1 for its guidelines.

The primary accessibility guidelines for webpages and applications are maintained by the World Wide Web Consortium (W3C), which is an international consortium that produces standards for web content. The guidelines relevant to websites are known as the Web Content Accessibility Guidelines, or WCAG. The current version of WCAG (as of June 2018) is WCAG 2.1, and it outlays 13 core principles of web content being perceivable, operable, understandable and robust (W3C 2018). Within those standards are a subset of testable "Success Criteria" which determine level of accessibility for those broader guidelines. There are three levels for criteria: A, AA, and AAA, with AAA being the highest. Most governmental laws and policies strive for a minimum of AA. For example, there is a principle that requires things to be "Operable" on a website, but within that principle, there are guidelines such as "Keyboard Accessible" and "Enough Time." Within a guideline such as "Keyboard Accessible" there would be success criterion for "Keyboard" (2.1.1) that states that all the content functionality must work from a keyboard (i.e., not just through a touch screen or mouse input).

There is a strong need for empirical data on the time impact on Blind users regarding accessibility barriers. This empirical data is necessary for understanding how much time is lost by Blind users, when they face specific barriers. This data is needed for both: (1) economic models used in regulations and (2) for future accessibility guidelines.

As governments around the world increase or clarify the requirements related to web accessibility for public accommodations, they often require some level of cost-benefit analysis for the proposed regulation (for instance, in the U.S., this is known as a regulatory impact analysis). As a part of these cost-benefit analyses, it's important to understand not only the costs of making technology accessible, but also the costs to Blind users (and people with other disabilities) of not making the technologies accessible.

This empirical data on the time lost due to accessibility barriers is also necessary for understanding that all of the success criteria within accessibility guidelines are not equal—compliance with some success criteria has a minor impact on users, while compliance with other success criteria has a major impact (and the impact may differ on what type of disability you have). So, quantifying time data on the disparity between high and low accessibility could potentially impact both future accessibility guidelines, as well as regulations. Furthermore, many public and private organizations fail to view web accessibility from a perspective that accounts for lost time and the resulting impact on worker productivity. When technologies aren't accessible for employees with disabilities, that time lost is a cost to the company. Significant time differences due to inaccessibility could negatively impact the ability of individuals to conduct tasks—for example, searching for public information, conducting financial transactions, and applying for employment. Government, researchers, developers, and disability advocates would benefit from some quantifiable estimates relating to the time disparities for Blind users between accessible and inaccessible web-based interfaces.

2 Background

In a 2007 study (Lazar et al. 2007), it was discovered that frustrating situations involving the use of the Web led to Blind users losing, on average, 30.4% of time. However, the amount of time lost exclusively due to accessibility barriers was not quantified. It is important to acknowledge that the definition of a "frustrating situation" can be misunderstood as a situation arising solely from web inaccessibility independent from other factors. While some of the problems that led to frustration and time lost were a result of inaccessibility encountered on web pages, there were frustrating and time-consuming problems related to poor performance of the assistive technology (AT) being used by the Blind users. There were also web pages users encountered that were fairly accessible but were not usable, so more time was needed to complete basic tasks. These problems included "(a) page layout causing confusing screen reader feedback; (b) conflict between screen reader and application; (c) poorly designed/unlabeled forms; (d) no alt text for pictures; and (e) 3-way tie between misleading links, inaccessible PDF, and a screen reader crash" (Lazar et al. 2007). In 2017, the U.S. Access Board Final Regulatory Impact Analysis for the updated version of Sect. 508 cited the 2007 study conducted by Lazar et al. as support for the notion that web accessibility causes time lost for Blind users. The text from the regulatory impact analysis is as follows:

> *"Lazar et al. (*2007*) find that blind participants reported losing, on average, 30.4% of time spent on the computer due to the frustration with situations from inaccessible/unusable web pages and AT malfunctions. Other studies reached similar conclusions".*
>
> (U.S. Access Board 2017)

Although it is true that those situations contributed to frustration and time lost, it would not be accurate to say that the frustration and time lost experienced by users was solely due to the inaccessibility encountered on the Web. Rather, the frustration arose from some situations of inaccessibility, but also screen reader crashes, screen reader incompatibility, poor formatting, and other factors related to AT and not solely the Web. The 2017 U.S. Access Board Final Regulatory Impact Analysis also mentions a 2004 study conducted by the Disability Rights Commission – "The Web: Access & Inclusion for Disabled People." The Disability Rights Commission conducted this research to formally investigate various shortcomings involving web inaccessibility and policy that should enforce accessibility. A segment of the investigation included a controlled study that observed task and time performance of Blind users and sighted users on websites with low accessibility and high accessibility. The purpose of this portion of the investigation was to identify barriers to accessibility for people with disabilities and then help develop solutions for them. The recorded results indicated that even on high accessibility websites, the Blind users needed more time to complete a task than sighted users. However, it was also concluded that "both blind users and non-impaired users took far longer on low accessibility sites than on high accessibility sites, and that this effect was not much more pronounced for disabled users…" (Disability Rights Commission 2004). While the studies conducted by Lazar et al. and the Disability Rights Commission both yield results involving time lost by Blind users on the web, neither study had the primary focus of determining how web accessibility barriers exclusively impact the time it takes Blind users to complete a task.

The idea that Blind users spend more time on the Web than other users due to accessibility barriers is not a novel one. In 2010 research by Babu et al. (2010) barriers faced by users in the context of accessibility and usability were studied. A portion of the study involved observing Blind users responding to short answer questions when navigating to an input field. They found that "the user's productivity is adversely affected due to the time and effort spent identifying the input field" because the input fields were not entirely compliant with "the understandability factor" of WCAG. While the study did find a situation in which an accessibility barrier caused Blind users to spend extra time on a task, the time was not quantified, and the study also considered usability barriers not directly caused by WCAG noncompliance. Additionally, in a 2007 study by Bigham et al. (2007) the behaviors of Blind users and their time spent browsing the Web were recorded. Bigham concluded that the Blind users "took more time to access all pages than their sighted counterparts." However, Bigham's analysis did not quantify the time spent on specific tasks with accessibility barriers due exclusively to WCAG violations.

Although the aforementioned studies did not quantify time spent or lost by Blind users in tasks, a different study conducted by Watanabe in 2009 quantified the task completion time of Blind and sighted users on controlled websites. One of the websites included properly labelled headings, and the other did not. After analyzing the data, it was concluded that Blind users had a decreased task completion time when headings were properly labelled. Watanabe explains that "for task 1, some of the blind subjects spent about 20 to 40 s to navigate through the structured site, while they typically spent from 60 to 70 s to navigate through the unstructured site." Even though the task completion time was decreased for Blind users, Wantanabe states "blind subjects tend to take about twice as long to complete a task for both structured and unstructured sites."

The conclusions from Watanabe's 2009 research are relevant, but they do not entirely encapsulate all time lost due to accessibility barriers. WCAG Success Criterion 2.4.6 states that in order for a website to be accessible to level AA, "Headings and labels describe topic or purpose" (W3C 2018). However, it was noted in the study that the controlled websites were entirely accessible when the heading variable was not considered. While Watanabe's study revealed time data that quantified the time spent by Blind users on controlled, static websites with one specific accessibility barrier, it does not provide a comprehensive understanding of how much time is lost by Blind users due exclusively to WCAG violations in a less controlled, dynamic setting that is much more representative of the websites Blind users access regularly.

3 Research Methods

When doing research involving users with disabilities, there are multiple methodological issues to consider, such as the sample size (typically smaller than for more general populations), material format (e.g. audio, large print, or braille?), and distribution of participants geographically (if there aren't enough users with a specific disability nearby, whether you should do remote research) (Lazar et al. 2017). One of the most important methodological considerations is whether you should utilize a user's own technical environment, with their own assistive technologies and settings, or use a consistent technology environment, which is identical and used for all participants.

3.1 Potential Research Methodologies

For users with disabilities, when you utilize a user's own technology, it documents the optimal performance of the users, because the user's setup has already been designed around the needs of that specific user (Lazar et al. 2017). All of the settings (e.g., screen reader rate of speech, chosen voice) are maximized to what a user needs. At the same time, it means that the technical environment differs from user to user, and therefore may not be appropriate using some types of experimental design where you must control for the technology across all users. However, when the research design focuses on studying user behavior or performance, you don't need to control for technology used, because you "want" to measure users at their best performance level, with other factors being controlled for (Lazar et al. 2017). For the current study, where we want to measure user performance when users encounter various barriers, it is appropriate to have users utilizing their own technologies, so that the data collected will be conservative and appropriate.

The core methodological approach of the current study is to have users attempt identical tasks, one on a high accessibility website, and one on a low accessibility site, and compare the time differences. Note that we describe it differently from the common terms "accessible" and "inaccessible." If a site is completely inaccessible, tasks cannot be completed by users with disabilities due to accessibility barriers. Yet just saying, "it's inaccessible" does not give any useful data, since the time to complete a task would either be zero or infinity (depending on how you frame the inability to complete a task, but that's more of a philosophical argument). So it's necessary to compare high accessibility sites (with no or minimal barriers) to low accessibility sites, where there are accessibility barriers but the tasks can still be completed. Since the goal is to collect data that can be utilized in policy, we must be sensitive to the fact that we need to create tasks that users can complete. We can't simply create tasks that result in users giving up on every task (even though we are aware that some users will give up on some tasks), because that doesn't get us to the data that are needed for regulatory impact analysis, even if that might be acceptable for a typical usability test.

There is another question to be considered regarding control of the test environment. Ideally, we want to have users interacting with existing, live websites, because that would be most representative of the actual amount of time lost due to low accessibility websites. However, it's unknown if there are simply too many uncontrollable factors in live websites. For instance, while sites can be evaluated for low accessibility and high accessibility, it's unknown if there are too many uncontrollable variables, and whether creating simple sites with simple interactions (and without extraneous factors), would be better.

Therefore, this research had two potential methodological approaches, both of which will be evaluated through the use of pilot studies, to determine which is the most effective. The first approach that we completed was to use existing, "live" websites, which after evaluation are deemed to be either low accessibility or high accessibility. The other approach is to use very basic website structures, created from scratch for the study, which remove the various confounding factors from the existing sites (using an approach similar to Hochheiser and Lazar in 2010).

3.2 Pilot Study for Approach One: Using Existing, "Live" Sites

The websites for the pilot study were selected as sites that would fall under the purview of the 12 categories of public accommodations per the U.S. Title III of the Americans with Disabilities Act. It was decided that category 1 (places of lodging), category 2 (establishments serving food and drink), category 6 (service establishments, including health care providers), and category 10 (places of education) would be used as a sample of the categories for site selection. Then, within the four categories, a significant number of websites were inspected for WCAG compliance and violations to determine both high and low accessibility sites for each. As noted previously, the low accessibility sites had the additional challenge of trying to ensure that the level of inaccessibility would not prevent users from being able to complete tasks.

The pilot testing included a total of five participants, four females and one male, ranging in age from 22 to 64. Each participant had at least five years of experience using a screen reader and the average for screen reader experience is 19.8 years. Four out of the five participants use JAWS as their primary screen reader, while the remaining participant uses VoiceOver as their primary screen reader (as noted earlier, the participants all used their own technologies maximized with their own settings). Participant experience with the Web/Internet ranged from 10 years to 30 years, with the average being 19 years of experience on the Web/Internet. Each of the five participants has some college experience. One participant is currently a sophomore undergraduate student, two participants are college graduates, one participant has a Master's degree, and one participant has both a Master's degree and a PhD.

The task list was chosen after careful consideration of the accessibility barriers present on each website, and also with regards to what would be considered a representative user task. Each task type also had to be equally replicated across all of the websites in a category. So, if one grocery website had a data retrieval task, then all of the grocery store websites needed to support equal, but not identical, data retrieval tasks.

After completing a pilot study of approach one, we determined that approach one is not an effective method for obtaining the quantified time data for high versus low accessibility. After conducting the pilot studies and analyzing the results, we determined that there are often confounding factors on existing, "live" websites, and the necessary approach of using each individual user's device and assistive technology on the live sites further complicates clear time data. This approach cannot provide a distinct "high accessibility" versus "low accessibility" framework to use for quantitative analysis.

For example, one of the users thought that a website did not have an accessible "Find a Store" search, even though the button was accessible with regards to WCAG. The screen reader would say "Find a Store button", but if the user navigated to the element next to it, the screen reader would say "Search button". The sequence of those buttons created confusion for the user because they thought the "Search" button initiated the search for "Find a Store" button. What really happened was that the user was taken to a page that searches the entire website upon clicking the "Search" button, and they could not find the store address information they were looking for.

A second website example was a store that had an occasional pop-up dialog box regarding a current promotion. This may or may not be displayed to users during the collection of data, and when that pop-up was displayed, it could present a case where the task on the website could not be completed at all (even though this would otherwise be a task that should be able to generate time data).

4 Future Steps: Pilot Study for Approach Two

The next stage of this project will involve the preparation of two separate website structures that we will create solely for the project. One site will include high accessibility design practices, and the second site will include common accessibility barriers that are found on websites. We will then conduct a pilot study with Blind users to determine whether this methodology provides more concrete time data than the previously attempted methodological approach. If the pilot study shows promise in terms of collecting data, we will then begin a more expansive study with a larger number of users.

The eligibility of participants for the pilot study for approach two will be determined the same way as for approach one. The format of the pilot study for this approach will have a similar structure to the original pilot tests that have been completed. Using the websites that we created, participants will be instructed to complete representative user tasks in a high accessibility and a low accessibility setting. The time it takes the participant to complete each user task will be recorded, and then all of the time data will be analyzed to quantify how much time was lost due to the presence of accessibility barriers.

Acknowledgements. The work reported in this publication was supported, in part, by grant number 90RE5027 (Universal Interface & Information Technology Access RERC) and 90REGE0008 (Inclusive ICT RERC), from the National Institute on Disability, Independent Living, and Rehabilitation Research, U.S. Administration for Community Living, Department of Health and Human Services. Grantees undertaking projects with government sponsorship are encouraged to express freely their findings and conclusions. Points of view or opinions do not, therefore, necessarily represent official policy of the Federal government.

References

Babu R, Singh R, Ganesh J (2010) Understanding blind users' web accessibility and usability problems. AIS Trans Hum-Comput Interact 2(3):73–94

Bigham J, Cavender A, Brudvik J, Wobbrock J, Ladner R (2007) WebinSitu: a comparative analysis of blind and sighted browsing behavior. In: Proceedings of ASSETS 2007, Tempe, AZ, US, 14–17 October 2007

Bloomberg (2019) Supreme court won't hear Domino's Pizza website access dispute. news.bloomberglaw.com/tech-and-telecom-law/supreme-court-wont-hear-dominos-pizza-website-access-dispute. Accessed 7 Oct 2019

Disability Rights Commission (2004) The web: Access & inclusion for disabled people. disability-studies.leeds.ac.uk/wp-content/uploads/sites/40/library/DRC-Web-FI.pdf. Accessed 10 Oct 2019

EFTA (2014) Standard - EN 301 549. mandate376.standards.eu/standard. Accessed 9 Oct 2019

GEO (2015) Equality Act 2010: Guidance. www.gov.uk/guidance/equality-act-2010-guidance. Accessed 7 Oct 2019

Hochheiser H, Lazar J (2010) Revisiting breadth vs. depth in menu structures for blind users of screen readers. Interact Comput 22(5):389–398

Lazar J, Allen A, Kleinman J, Malarkey C (2007) What frustrates screen reader users on the web: a study of 100 blind users. Int J Hum-Comput Interact 22(3):247–269

Lazar J, Feng JH, Hochheiser H (2017) Research methods in human-computer interaction. Morgan Kaufmann/Elsevier, Cambridge

Lazar J, Goldstein DF, Taylor A (2015) Ensuring digital accessibility through process and policy. Morgan Kaufmann/Elsevier, Waltham

LF Legal (2019) Big win for web accessibility in Domino's Pizza case. www.lflegal.com/2019/01/dominos-ninth-circuit/?fbclid=IwAR17trrSpmvvPNi16D8R331AWfG1oRE5bU7HQEm1zAJdmW01_bHHEaScSbc. Accessed 23 Jan 2019

National Archives (2018) The public sector bodies (websites and mobile applications) (No. 2) Accessibility regulations 2018. www.legislation.gov.uk/uksi/2018/952/made. Accessed 7 Oct 2019

U.S. Access Board (2017) Final regulatory impact analysis. www.access-board.gov/guidelines-and-standards/communications-and-it/about-the-ict-refresh/final-regulatory-impact-analysis. Accessed 10 Oct 2019

Watanabe T (2009) Experimental evaluation of usability and accessibility of heading elements. Disabi Rehabil Assistive Technol 4(4): 236–247

W3C (2018) Web content accessibility guidelines. www.w3.org/TR/WCAG21/. Accessed 5 Oct 2019

Thinking Bias: The Hidden Talent Excluder

A. Burns[1(✉)], R. Davies[1], and P. M. Langdon[2]

[1] Catapult Solutions Ltd., Gillingham, Dorset, UK
{andreaburns,richard.davies}@catapult-solutions.co.uk
[2] Cambridge Engineering Design Centre, University of Cambridge, Cambridge, UK
pml24@cam.ac.uk

Abstract. Large numbers of organisations use interviews and psychometric tests as methods of recruiting new employees. The inherent biases of these approaches are examined here for a number of common scenarios and the implications for inclusivity explored. Axiology or Value Science has been proposed as a philosophy and approach that analyses and leverages the concept of value judgement and provides practical methods by which it can be deployed to reduce organisational bias and increase inclusion via identifying, leveraging and raising the levels of cognitive diversity within organisations. In particular, the methods of Axiometrics are examined and contrasted with those of psychometrics; along with a detailed look at its validation in practice. It concludes that Axiometrics is superior to personality and behavioural based psychometrics in fostering diversity and therefore effectiveness in organisations by increasing understanding of people capability.

1 The Hidden Diversity and Inclusivity Challenge

Traditionally, a large proportion of leaders and managers have tended to attract, recruit and retain talent in their own image. This interviewer bias is known as the Similarity Bias. This states that individuals get along with people who tend to look and think like we do. If both the interviewer and interviewee are similar, whether in demographics or even education level, they will develop more accurate perceptions of the other's self-concepts, as the two self-concepts will be similar (Sears and Rowe 2003). A more accurate perception and validation to the interviewer's self-concept by the interviewee would lead to higher interview ratings and scores. This phenomenon is either conscious or unconscious.

This bias doesn't end with the recruiting process. Colleagues gravitate toward the people who think and express themselves in a similar way. As a result, organisations often end up with like-minded teams. When this happens, we have what psychologists call functional bias; and low cognitive diversity (Govindarajan and Gupta 2002). This is a matter for concern since similarity and functional bias can have the consequent effect of excluding people from the workplace – simply because they think differently.

Today, most progressive leaders attempt to counteract conscious and unconscious bias and take steps to build diverse teams and cultures that embrace diversity. They strive to hit the right balance of gender and ethnicity. They are inclusive of people with disabilities and respect all sexual orientations. Despite the progress made in the last three decades, recent studies demonstrate the significant cost to industry of the lack of

P. Langdon et al. (Eds.): CWUAAT 2020, *Designing for Inclusion*, pp. 161–172, 2020.
https://doi.org/10.1007/978-3-030-43865-4_17

diversity. Frost (2014), Head of Diversity and Inclusion for the 2012 London Olympic Games, states that "discrimination against women, homosexuals and disabled people is estimated to cost $64bn a year in the US alone".

Deloitte's (2011) report says: "it is not enough to create a corporate version of Noah's Ark bringing in "two of each kind". Once a diverse team has been assembled, the way each person is treated must be inclusive – respecting and recognising each person's value and diversity (Liswood 2009).

More needs to be done to improve diversity. But there's a deeper and more costly diversity problem. A hidden diversity crisis. In general, scant consideration is given to the diversity of thinking patterns across team members. The reason for this gap is simple. It has not been easy, or affordable to recognise cognitive traits with accuracy. The way in which people think, is a way to predict how they will perform. When members of a team think in the same way, they are open to common blind spots. They miss the challenge from people who think and see things differently. As a result, the quality of decision making suffers (Peck and Levashina 2017). Poor decision-making leads to poor performance. This lack of recognition and appreciation of different thinking patterns is a contributing factor to Groupthink.

Groupthink is a psychological phenomenon born of our innate desire to conform with others. First coined in 1972 the term specifically refers to the tendency for a group to make bad or poorly thought-out decisions because its members aligned themselves with one another, insulating themselves from outside opinion and reinforcing viewpoints they already share (Turner and Pratkanis 1998).

Groupthink can cause serious problems. For example, it may have been a significant contributor to the banking practices that led to the global economic collapse of 2008–2009. The driving belief was that housing prices would continue to rise, no matter what. Groupthink may have pushed banks to extend themselves more and more. The banks perceived it to be smarter to stay within the confines of the philosophy and actions of the group. This drove the housing market to collapse (Atiyas et al. 2013).

1.1 Addressing the Hidden Diversity Gap

Deborah Dehaas, Vice Chair, Center for Corporate Governance, and Chief Inclusion Officer at Deloitte LLP, sums up the benefits from diversity in thinking styles:

> *"Embedding diversity of thought – as well as diversity of people – is a healthy way to challenge the status quo and help directors view issues through a new lens. Granted, introducing diverse ideas to the boardroom is not always comfortable. There's value in the added perspective as it enriches the conversation and provides board members with a fresh point of view."*
>
> (Dehaas 2015)

Clive Hyland writes in People Management:

> *"Any human performance strategy – whether individual, team or organisational – needs to draw the best from each of the three brain regions (cortex, limbic and basal) if it is to unlock our true potential. In practical terms, this means:*

- *Having the right 'machinery' in place*
- *Ensuring appropriate relationships are sustained*
- *Most crucially, working to establish a believable vision"*

(Hyland 2017)

Any diversity and inclusivity strategy should involve accurate and objective assessment of an individual's ability across these areas of the brain – irrespective of age, gender, ethnicity or disability. What is needed is an objective approach that can identify thinking patterns and diversity of thinking, irrespective of the body it comes in. Axiology (Hartman 1967) is a scientific methodology that does just this.

1.2 The Definition and Origins of Axiology

Axiology is the science of value. The word Axiology is derived from two Greek roots 'axios' (which means value) and 'logos' (theory) – hence it is the theory of value. There are two different and distinct areas of axiology, the **philosophical** and the **formal**. Aristotle can be regarded as the father of philosophical axiology.

1.3 Formal Axiology – Value Mathematics

Dr Robert S. Hartman (1910–1973) is regarded as the father of modern value science or Formal Axiology. He theorised that the primary difference between natural order and moral disorder lay in the mathematics which orders the natural world. He discovered that all value has scientific order based on transfinite mathematical sets. In doing so, he identified the principles which may order and structure not only our moral decisions, but all our value judgements. There are applications in psychology, sociology, psychiatry, law, theology, political science, finance, and decision theory.

1.4 Foundations of Formal Axiology

According to Hartman's system "value" is a phenomena or concept, and the value of anything is determined by the extent to which it meets the intent of its meaning. For example, a chair that has all of the natural properties contained within the definition of chair is by definition a "good chair." A chair that has only a few of the natural properties contained within the definition of a chair is by definition a "less than good" or "not as good" chair, a fair chair, a poor chair, etc.

A "good chair," according to Hartman, fulfils the intention of its definition. Given that premise, Hartman's theories set forth a system of mathematics to establish and prove the accuracy and utility of his theories.

Hartman discovered that every concept has three dimensions and that every concept has the following types of value:

1. The value of its uniqueness.
2. The value of its function or role.
3. The value of its meaning and purpose.

These three "Dimensions of Value" are referred to as the following concepts:

1. Intrinsic Value—the capacity for discerning values concerning uniqueness and individuality.
2. Extrinsic Value—the capacity for discerning role, function and practicality.
3. Systemic Value—the capacity for discerning values concerning meaning, purpose, order and system.

1.4.1 Three Value Dimensions – The World and the Self

Hartman developed a tool to understand and report on human thinking and evaluation. He realised we actually apply the three value dimensions in two ways:

- Everything we see outside of ourselves he called **The World**
- Everything relating to our inner thinking he referred to as **The Self**

Figure 1 shows the three value dimensions across World and Self View.

1.4.2 Hartman's Three Dimensions of Value

Let's illustrate the difference between these three dimensions of value by using each one to describe a smartphone.

- *Intrinsic Value*: The smartphone signifies to the world that you are part of modern society, you want to stay in touch with your friends, share your life with them, comment on their lives. You cherish the satisfaction of getting a status update and playing the latest games with friends. You feel lost without your smartphone
- *Extrinsic Value*: This smartphone is an item of communication, value £500, beveled edges, sized to fit your palm, shiny colour
- *Systemic Value*: The smartphone is a communications device based on cellular radio technology.

2 Link to Brain Regions and the Three Dimensions

2.1 The Single Axiological Norm

Hartman's approach was not based on observation of behaviour or personality as is the case with psychometric profiling tools. He deduced and then proved that the structure of thought has its own single norm. This norm is inclusive. It has been proven to be the same for people all over the world, regardless of culture, race, income, age, gender, or other factors – we all have the same structure of thought (Hartman 1967). It is a proven scientific tool that can be used to combat bias and foster inclusivity. Hartman did not create inductive norms by observing and correlating behaviour, he scientifically validated his deduced value theory and confirmed a single objective norm that already exists in all of us. This evolved into The Hartman Value Profile (HVP). The HVP is made up of two 18-item inventories designed to measure values placed by subjects within the three dimensions of value.

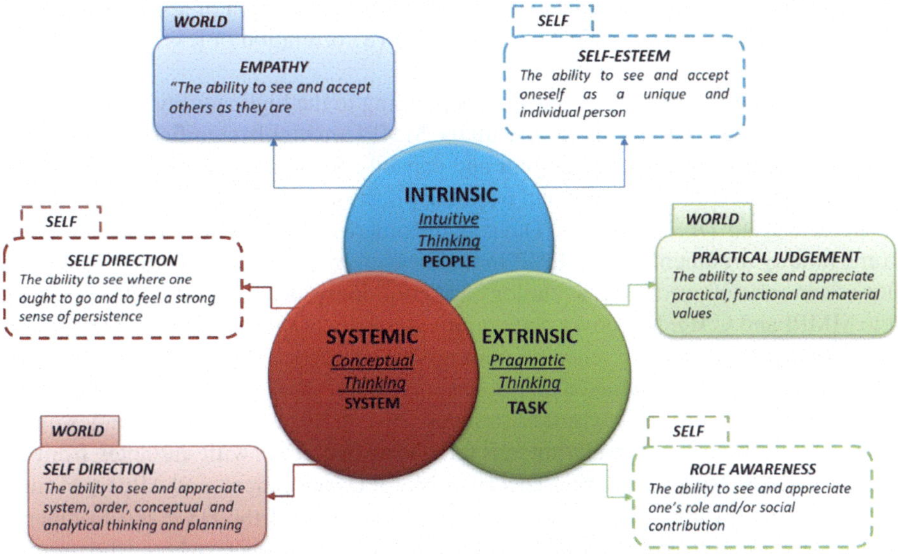

Fig. 1. The three dimensions of value – Catapult Solutions Ltd

2.2 How Reliable Is the Hartman Value Profile?

The instrument reliability study of the HVP (HVPI and II) was a study performed by Value Resource Group (Axiometrics International Inc. 2002). The reliability of an instrument measured the probability that the results of the assessments generated by the instrument are not a result of chance. This study analysed Hartman scores. Two samples used in this analysis were selected from an applicant database generated for Dollar General Corporation (large Retailers in the USA) over a three-year test project. Two hundred re-test situations were used for the reliability analysis. The 200 profiles used were selected in random from a larger population of approximately 6 000 applicants re-tested at different times.

Both sets of data were evaluated with the Spearman Rank Order Correlation Analysis and the results provided correlation at a confidence level of $p < .001$. In the raw scores analysis the correlation coefficients were greater than .549. The final rank order coefficient was .974, indicating "an extremely high level of significance and confidence in the reliability of the instrument, which is far greater in significance than provided by a $p < .001$".

A comparative analysis of the HVP and the Minnesota Multiphasic personality inventory MMPI was conducted by Dr. Leon Pomeroy (Davis and Pomeroy 1982), Director of the Behavioral Medicine Unit at the Veterans Affairs (VA) Outpatient Clinic in Brooklyn,

New York, US. Results showed that one hundred and twenty eight (128) HVP/MMPI item had a correlation of less than $p < .05$, and (75) had a correlation of better than $p < .001$.

- The PBI/HVP correlation indicated 18 scores with a correlation of less than $p < .05$
- The CMI/HVP correlation indicated 6 scores with a correlation of less than $p < .05$
- The AL/HVP correlation indicated 4 scores with a correlation of less than $p < .05$.

These are highly significant correlations pointing to the high validity for the HVP in clinical applications. The correlations with the MMPI are highly significant and indicate that the measure of one's value system and capacity for making value judgments is a significant measure that has valid and useful applications.

The data from Dr. Pomeroy's (Davis and Pomeroy 1982) studies establish a concurrent validity argument for the HVP in the measurement of self-defeating behavioral states commonly referred to as psychology and commonly measured by such instruments as the MMPI and CAQ. Moreover, the empirical results of the study provide credibility for the HVP, as well as the science of axiology itself.

Dr. John Austin has conducted additional correlation studies on the value of the HVP for education to identify highly gifted students. He conducted a series of studies on the measure of moral value, correlating variables from the HVP with variables from the Rokeach Value Survey, Kohlberg's Theory of Moral Development, and Allport-Vernon-Lindzey Study of Values. The correlations from his study of the HVP and Kohlberg's moral variables and Rokeach variables show a higher significance (where Rho, or measure of statistical correlation was largely above .900) than the variables from the study of specific values from the Allport et al. study. These results are to be expected, since the HVP measures one's capacity to make value judgments rather than the measure of one's specific values (Axiometrics International Inc. 2002).

2.3 From Hartman Value Profile to Axiometrics

Since the early 1970s, Professor Carpenter (1991) focused on developing and validating a computerised system of Axiological analysis. He produced his first computerised model in 1983. (A timeline of the key validation studies is available by request, email: value@axiometricspartners.com).

2.4 What Does Axiometrics Do?

Proponents suggest that it accurately measures cognitive processes and delivers a rich perspective in human behaviour. It does this ethically and with near-instant results. Axiometrics provides an unprecedented aid to understanding human capacities in individual, societal and organisational constructs. It identifies the values and valuing system upon which an individual bases their decisions. It identifies their skills, talent, "access to talent" and attitude within a specific environment. It gives a root cause understanding of behaviour and talent. It reveals aspects of their sub-conscious. The Axiometric technique enable neuroscientists, psychologists, anthropologists and others to understand why people do what they do using deductive rather than inductive methods that are used in Psychometrics.

2.5 Psychometric Inductive Methodology

Psychometric measurement is inductive, reasoning from the particular to the general. Items are collected, grouped through such methods as factor analysis, then assumed to measure actual traits, usually through self- or other report. Items within the groups are not theoretically connected – this must be considered when building diverse teams as true comparison of one individual with another is not possible due to the data not being a full analysis of the individuals decision-making capacity. One item in the group is assumed to measure the trait as much as the next one does. Thus a person could be considered to be extroverted if they agreed with any set of self-descriptors within the pool loading on the factor Extraversion.

2.6 Axiometric Deductive Methodology

Axiometric measurement is deductive – reasoning from the general to the particular. A person's actual thinking process is measured against a universal norm and specific traits identified. Deduction is logical, traits are organically related and derived through an "if-then" process. If a person weights their deviation from the universal algorithm in the direction of strategic thinking, we know they are a strategic thinker.

The Axiometrics deductive technique allows people to understand decision-forming and thinking process patterns quickly without the biases implicit in either self-reporting or observer behaviour and is consequently reliable and 'ungameable'. What do we mean by ungameable'? 'Gaming' is when people try to second guess profiling questions and provide the answers that they think will be most valued by the people who will be reviewing and making recruitment, development or promotion decisions based on the test results. This behaviour is not new. It is recognised in the well-known Hawthorne effect which recognises a type of reactivity in which individuals modify an aspect of their behaviour in response to their awareness of being observed (Mayo 1933). There is an associated ethical issue that has been created by the widespread practice of using psychometric profiling tools as a key tool in the recruitment process. Students are being trained to influence the outcome so that they do not come out as introverted – since that is deemed to reduce their changes of being hired (Turban et al. 2017).

In organisations, Axiometrics can be used to diagnose individual and team developmental needs. It can also be used to establish a departmental thinking pattern benchmark, i.e., a measurable definition of 'what good looks like for individuals' in, e.g., the sales, marketing, accounting or HR departments. This can then be used to assist recruitment by comparing candidates to the benchmark for a specific function. This takes the guesswork out of recruitment. Axiometrics can be used across the whole talent lifecycle from recruitment, onboarding, personal development, succession capability development, people risk analysis, team/board effectiveness. Axiometrics enables leaders, trainers and coaches to design developmental work assignments, appropriate training or coaching to help individuals and teams fulfill their potential. It can be used to help organisations define and develop their culture.

3 Axiometric and Diversity Validity

3.1 Equal Employment Opportunity Commission and Axiometrics

The fundamental principle underlying Federal Law and Regulation in pre-employment and career assessment practices is as follows:

> "*Employer policies and practices which have an adverse impact on the employment opportunities of any race, sex or ethnic group are illegal.*"
>
> (EEOC 1978)

In an effort to protect the rights of the citizens, the Equal Employment Opportunity Commission (EEOC) established three requirements for any testing instrument used as part of the hiring decision process:

- The instrument must measure what it says it measures
- The instrument cannot discriminate according to age, race, or sex
- Whatever the instrument measures must have a direct application to the position being applied for.

The third requirement is the responsibility of the hiring organisation to monitor. The other two are conditions of the instrument itself. The industry standard used for validating instruments for effectiveness and accuracy is the Minnesota Multi-Phasic Personality Inventory (MMPI). A 100% statistical concurrency between the MMPI and HVP, entitled "Concurrent Validity Study of Hartman's Valuemetrics and Value Science Assumptions as a Revolutionary New Basis for Modern Behavior Science Applications" was published in the VA practitioner by Dr. Leon Pomeroy and Dr. John Davis (Edwards and Davis 2014). Another study performed by Austin and Garwood (1976) was presented to the National Association of School Psychologists in March 1977 (Axiometrics International Inc. 2002). This study of the most prominent value measurement instruments validates the HVP in the measurement of value structures.

3.2 How Does Axiometrics Differ to Psychometrics?

Most psychometric assessments require users to complete a questionnaire. This is known as self-reporting. Another popular technique is to collate feedback from others – peers, direct reports and supervisors (i.e., a 360-degree report). As Dr. Robert Hogan of Hogan Assessments noted ATP Conference in Phoenix (2014), "self-report doesn't give an accurate picture of the person", hence the preoccupation when controlling "faking" (Donaldson and Grant-Vallone 2002). Moreover, as Hogan (2014) also mentioned, self-knowledge can be an issue. He stated that "the only people who really know themselves are the psychologists".

The words 'test' and 'measurement', as used in psychology, are misleading because of the implied similarity to scientific measurements. Conventional psychological testing is quite different from scientific measurements in natural sciences. Psychological measurement is an estimation of a psychological construct (Michell 1997). Psychological and personality, intelligence, attitude and motivation tests are different from quantitative measurements in physical sciences such as height and weight. As Kline (2000), Professor of Psychometrics, Exeter University, said:

> *"There are no units of [psychological] measurement and no true zeros. Whatever psychological measurement is, it is not scientific measurement as defined in natural sciences... If we consider what is meant by intelligence or extraversion, just for example, it is by no means clear what units of measurement might be used or what the true zero may mean. This problem applies to the majority of psychological concepts and variables."*
>
> (Kline 2000)

It is often mistakenly believed that psychological tests are 'objective', meaning that their findings and scores reflect an outside existence and are real or approximate something close to it. The term objectivity has an entirely different meaning when applied to psychological tests or measurements. It refers to the standard ways in which they are administered, recorded and interpreted.

3.3 How Does Axiometrics Differ to Psychometrics When It Comes to Recruiting Effective Teams?

A Harvard Business Review (HBR) paper reported the findings of a study by Schmidt and Hunter (1998) that set out to discover the most effective recruitment selection processes and to reveal the practices that don't work as well. It was based on validity coefficients ranging from 0 to 1. The higher the number, the higher the correlation between test scores and predicted future job performance – see below.

Psychometrics personality tests typically using the Likert Scale or are Ipsative in assessment technique. They rank near the bottom – with a coefficient of only up to 0.22.

"There is little evidence of enduring relationships between personality test scores and measures of success at work" (Blinkhorn and Johnson 1990).

Axiometrics, on the other hand, is a cognitive ability test – these have a coefficient of 0.65. The top-ranking test is defined as 'multi-measure' which is a combination of cognitive ability, personality and interests (Fig. 2).

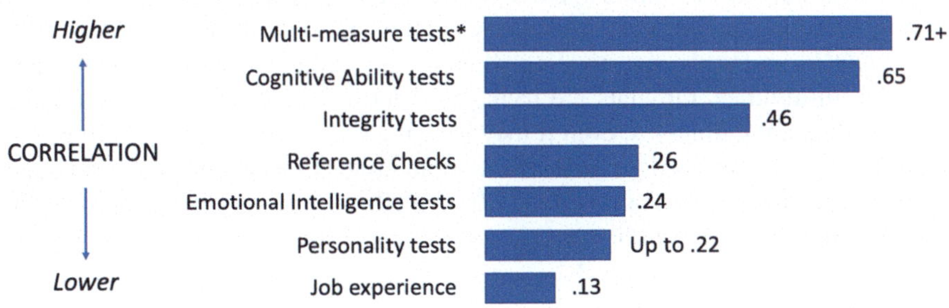

Fig. 2. The effectiveness of recruitment selection processes. Source based on data shared by Schmidt in an address to PTCMW (6 Nov 2013) as an update to Schmidt and Hunter (1998)

3.4 Further Differences – Axiometrics vs. Psychometrics

Axiometric assessment does not use self-reporting questionnaires to ask people to consciously describe themselves via a series of questions. With Axiometrics, people are required to take a 15-min online thinking exercise. This involves clicking and dragging two groups of 18 short phrases from most to least preferred. The thinking process they use to rank the phrases is tracked – using algorithms which have been developed over the past 40 years. There are 6.4 quadrillion variations of output. Psychometrics only work in the conscious. Psychometric profiling tools only gather information from self-reporting and observation. By definition, this is superficial.

3.4.1 Self-report Assessments Label People

We now return to two points mentioned earlier to consider the implications:

- Often people do not know themselves well
- There is strong pressure for presenting a positive picture of one-self in hiring/promotion situations (Donaldson and Grant-Vallone 2002).

This is concerning. Many people do not know themselves well, they put their faith in a psychometric methodology, such as Myers Briggs, to find career path guidance based upon one of the sixteen labels of the Myers Briggs classification system (or rely on other personality and behavioural systems such as Insights or DISC). If they then find their 'natural' label does not fit, they feel unsure about their suitability. This is where faking takes place – when a candidate second guesses the questions and provide different answers to obtain the 'right' label for a job application. Until recently, people often took such tests well into the hiring process, and the results were considered along with interviews and past experience. As the hiring process gets more automated the tests are used earlier in the process to winnow applicants.

In Mischel (1968), Mischel found that empirical studies often failed to support the fundamental assumption of personality theory, that an individual's behaviour remained highly consistent across diverse situations. He cautioned that an individual's behaviour was highly dependent upon situational cues – shaped largely by the exigencies of a given situation and that the notion that individuals act in consistent ways across different situations, reflecting the influence of underlying personality traits, is a myth.

The EOOC is currently investigating whether personality tests discriminate against people with disabilities. Officials are trying to determine if the tests shut out people suffering from mental illnesses, even if they have the right skills for the job. In general, personality-testing firms disclose little information, saying their formulas are proprietary. For example, Kronos Inc. has opposed the EEOC's efforts in a civil lawsuit to force them to hand over their internal validity studies.

4 Conclusions

This paper has set out the dangers of self-reporting psychometric reports in that they introduce an extra set of labels into the workplace and run the risk of introducing a new form of discrimination. Few people would describe a person by their racial, ethnic or gender stereotypes, but many have no reservations explaining others' behaviour with a personality and behavioural typologies like Myers-Briggs Type Indicator, Insights and DISC ("She's such an 'INTJ'"). The authors have contended that psychometric reports are inaccurate and can't predict job performance. Personality classifications at best capture only a small amount of variance in behaviour, and in combination only explain tangential aspects of dynamics in the workplace. Personality tests cannot measure inner experiences.

Organisations should instead focus on understanding cognitive traits, thinking styles and decision making. A lack of cognitive diversity reduces the opportunity to strengthen decision making by failing to enlist input from people who think differently. It also leads to unconscious bias that excludes talent.

We recommend recruitment and development processes should identify thinking difference and encourage cognitive diversity. When organisations face a new, uncertain, complex situation, they should build and deploy a team that has a spread of diverse thinking patterns. The authors advocate that inclusivity of different thinking patterns will be beneficial for all stakeholders. The ability to accurately measure cognitive process delivers a rich perspective in human behaviour. To do so ethically and with near-instant results provides us with an unprecedented aid to understanding human capacities. Axiometrics techniques enable neuroscientists, psychologists, and others to understand '*why people do what they do*' using deductive rather than inductive methods. It allows users to get to decision-forming and thinking process data quickly without biases in self-reporting or observer behaviour and is, consequently, reliable. More organisations must recognise and utilise diversity of thinking.

References

Atiyas I, Bhorat H, Dervis K, Drysdale P, Frischtak CR et al (2013) Think tank 20: the g-20 and central banks in the new world of unconventional monetary policy. Brookings, Washington, D.C.

Austin J, Garwood B (1976) The relationship of the Hartman value profile (HVP), the Rokeach value survey (RVS), Allport-Vernon-Lindzey study of values (AVL) and Kohlberg's theory of moral development (KMD): a series of axiometric studies, (Parts 1 and 2). Presented at the National Association of School Psychologists Convention, Cincinnati, US, March 1977

Axiometrics International Inc. (2002) Axiometrics™ validity studies of Hartman profile model. Revised 2019. www.axiometricspartners.com/images/ContentPDFs/ValidityWhitePapers/Axiometrics_Validity_Studies_prepared_by_Axiometrics_International_Inc_revised_2019.pdf. Accessed 1 Aug 2019

Blinkhorn S, Johnson C (1990) Nature 348(6303):671–672

Carpenter W (1991) Why good people do bad things. In: Edwards RB, Davis JW (eds) Forms of value and valuation: theory and applications. University Press of America, Lanham, MD, US. Republished 2014 by Wipf and Stock, Eugene, OR, US (1991, 2014)

Davis JW, Pomeroy LR (1982) Introduction to behavioural axiology, Part 1: a concurrent validity study of Hartman's valuemetrics and value science assumptions as a revolutionary new basis for modern behavioural science application. In: Proceedings of the 2nd international conference on the Cattell 16PF test. Institute for Personality and Aptitude Testing, Inc., Champaign, IL, US

Dehaas D (2015) Unleashing valuable new perspective in the boardroom. The Financier, May 2015. www.financierworldwide.com/unleashing-valuable-new-perspectives-in-the-boardroom/#.XXZkGShKhPY. Accessed 11 Sept 2019

Deloitte (2011) Only skin deep? Re-examining the business case for diversity. www.ced.org/pdf/Deloitte_-_Only_Skin_Deep.pdf. Accessed 15 Dec 2019

Donaldson SI, Grant-Vallone EJ (2002) Understanding self-report bias in organizational behavior research. J Bus Psychol 17:245–260

Edwards RB, Davis JW (2014) Forms of value and valuation: theory and applications. Wipf and Stock, Eugene

EEOC (1978) Equal Employment Opportunities Commission. For historical purposes, the original text of the law, without any subsequent amendments. www.eeoc.gov/eeoc/history/35th/thelaw/civil_service_reform-1978.html. Accessed 20 Jan 2020

Frost S (2014) The inclusion imperative: how real inclusion creates better business and builds better societies: courage, creativity and talent. Kogan Page, London

Govindarajan V, Gupta AK (2002) Building an effective global business team. IEEE Eng Manage Rev 30(2):28

Hartman RS (1967) The structure of value: foundations of scientific axiology. Southern Illinois University Press, Carbondale

Hogan R (2014) Personality theory and assessment: predicting career success and organizational effectiveness. Presented at innovations in testing conference. Association of Test Publishers (ATP), Scottsdale, AZ, US, 2–5 March 2014

Hyland C (2017) The neuro edge: people insights for leaders and practitioners. Panoma Press, St Albans

Kline P (2000) Handbook of psychological testing, 2nd edn. Routledge, London

Liswood LA (2009) the loudest duck: moving beyond diversity while embracing differences to achieve success at work. Wiley, New Jersey

Mayo GE (1933) Human problems of an industrial civilization. Macmillan Co., New York

Michell J (1997) Quantitative science and the definition of measurement in psychology. Br J Psychol 88(3):355–383

Mischel W (1968) Personality and assessment. Wiley, New York

Peck JA, Levashina J (2017) Impression management and interview and job performance ratings: a meta-analysis of research design with tactics in mind. Front Psychol 8:201

Schmidt FL, Hunter JE (1998) The validity and utility of selection methods in personnel psychology: practical and theoretical implications of 85 years of research findings. Psychol Bull 124(2):262–274

Sears GJ, Rowe PM (2003) A personality-based similar-to-me effect in the employment interview: conscientiousness, affect-versus competence-mediated interpretations, and the role of job relevance. Can J Behav Sci 35(1):13–24

Turban DB, Moake TR, Wu SYH, Cheung YH (2017) Linking extroversion and proactive personality to career success: the role of mentoring received and knowledge. J Career Dev 44(1):20–33

Turner ME, Pratkanis AR (1998) Twenty-five years of groupthink theory and research: lessons from the evaluation of a theory. Organ Behav Hum Decis Process 73(2–3):105–115

Improving PDF Accessibility Tools for Content Developers: Looking Towards the Future

A. Jembu Rajkumar(✉), J. B. Jordan, and J. Lazar

Trace Center, HCIL, College of Information Studies, University of Maryland, College Park, USA
{aravind,jbjordan,jlazar}@umd.edu

Abstract. While much of the discussion on digital accessibility focuses on web accessibility, accessibility of PDF files is an ongoing but frequently overlooked challenge. The guidelines for PDF accessibility, known as PDF Universal Accessibility (PDF U/A or the Matterhorn Protocol), are nowhere near as well known as the Web Content Accessibility Guidelines (WCAG). One of the greatest challenges is the insufficient level of tools to assist content creators. In a previous research paper was published in January 2020 (Jembu Rajkumar et al. 2020), our team used surveys, usability testing and interviews, to understand the challenges that content creators in STEM fields face in making PDF files accessible. In this paper, we propose next steps in tool development for improving PDF accessibility in the future.

1 Introduction

The primary purpose of the PDF format originally was to enable anyone to capture documents from any application, send electronic versions of these documents anywhere, and view and print them on any machine. This lets the content creator convert images, webpages and other content to generate standardised PDFs. Hence, PDF documents are essentially digital papers which are being used extensively in all spaces - governmental, industrial and educational. Today, the capabilities of PDF go beyond digital paper enabling the user to secure the documents with password protection, e-signatures, and version controlling. There are various content authoring tools like Microsoft Word, LaTeX, InDesign, and scripts by Google and Python which can create PDF files. With so many different ways to generate a PDF document, users may not know if they have generated an accessible PDF. A report says that there are approximately 2.5 trillion PDF documents available online, but it is unknown how many of those are accessible (Itext 2019).

According to the World Health Organization (WHO), there are about 253 million people who have some form of visual impairment (WHO 2018). These individuals usually rely upon assistive technologies such as screen readers. PDF documents that are not properly marked up or tagged are inaccessible to these users because screen readers may not read them in proper order or allow for efficient navigation. In order for a PDF to be accessible, both the content and the document's underlying structure must be free from issues that would alter or block information to users with disabilities. The document's underlying structure is known as the tag structure and it allows assistive technology

P. Langdon et al. (Eds.): CWUAAT 2020, *Designing for Inclusion*, pp. 173–181, 2020.
https://doi.org/10.1007/978-3-030-43865-4_18

(AT) users a way to interpret the content of the document in the same manner of a sighted user. Previous studies document that people with visual impairments describe inaccessible PDF documents as one of the greatest barriers to consuming digital content (Lazar et al. 2007; Tomlinson et al. 2016).

The technical specification for the PDF document's underlying structure is defined by a set of guidelines known as PDF Universal accessibility (PDF U/A). It consists of 31 checkpoints and 136 failure conditions which ensures accessibility in PDF documents who use assistive technologies including screen readers. Compliance to this set of conditions are either pass or fail unlike WCAG which has three levels of conformance. The concepts in WCAG apply to PDF documents, however, there is a level of interpretation needed to convert the WCAG concepts into the specific technical challenges of PDF documents; PDF/UA provides guidance more specific to PDF documents.

2 Previous Studies on PDF Accessibility

A study on the accessibility of academic papers in major accessibility or disability related conferences between 2009 to 2013 found out that 95.5% of the documents were untagged. Only 3% of the papers had alternate text for graphical content. 13.7% of the papers had title metadata. The author sampled around 200 papers and evaluated against 11 criteria by WCAG 2.0, though PDF/UA would have been a better fit (Nganji 2015).

Similarly, another study compared the accessibility of academic papers from ASSETS, CHI and W4A conference proceedings (Brady et al. 2015). CHI was the least accessible of the three conferences in 2014, although 2014 was the highest level of paper accessibility for CHI over a 6-year period, due to specific actions taken by the program committee (Lazar et al. 2017). ASSETS consistently had a higher percentage of paper accessibility, as it is a requirement for authors. After W4A introduced guidelines to make PDFs accessible in 2011, the number of tagged documents rose to 100% in 2014 (Brady et al. 2015).

In our previous research on tools for helping content creators make accessible PDF files (Jembu Rajkumar et al. 2020), there were two major findings. First, there was a lack of general awareness regarding PDF accessibility. To make a PDF completely accessible, there are various conditions that need to be satisfied such as specifying the language and title of the document, providing a proper reading order, having appropriate heading levels, alternate texts for images, accessible links etc., just to name a few. Participants who knew about PDF accessibility reported that they did just one or two of the above-mentioned conditions and assumed they made the document accessible. In addition, participants often confused being able to access a PDF (as in having the ability to find, download, and read the document) with accessible PDFs (that are accessible to people with disabilities). Many publishers do not ask authors to make their PDF files accessible and do not have detailed information on accessibility in the paper templates.

The second overall finding is that, even if people were aware of PDF accessibility, they felt they lacked the knowledge and tools to make accessible PDFs. Most tools that help to remediate accessibility issues are not open source and are often paid versions. These tools are not user friendly, let alone bug-free. There are some tools that check for accessibility issues and tell the content contributor where problems exist, but fewer tools help in remediating the accessibility barriers. Many participants in previous studies (Bigham et al. 2016; Jembu Rajkumar et al. 2020) have expressed that they are unhappy with the current tools that exist. Participants in our study also mentioned that these tools are quite complex to use, which makes it more difficult for content contributors to produce accessible documents. The biggest demotivation mentioned for not making accessible documents is the time that it takes or that it is perceived to take to make an accessible document (Jembu Rajkumar et al. 2020). Due to this reason, the majority of study participants felt that publishers should take the responsibility of making the PDF document accessible.

3 Our Vision for the Future of Tools

Effective tools are the broken link in improving PDF accessibility. What most individuals don't realise is that different content generation tools have different levels of accessibility markup when converted to PDF document. For instance, when creating a PDF file using Adobe Acrobat Pro from a Word document on a Mac, more accessibility markup will be present than when creating a PDF file directly using the current version of MS Word for Mac. The operating system in which the tool is hosted also plays a role in transferring the markup when converting a file to a PDF format. Windows and Macintosh operating systems have different ways of preserving the markup from various content authoring tools. While the metadata transfer from these tools to PDF is somewhat successful in the Windows operating system, that claim cannot be made for the Mac OS.

Making a document accessible is a two-part process. The first part is to identify the various PDF accessibility issues. The second part is to remediate these accessibility issues. Currently, there are various open source and free tools that help in identifying various accessibility issues including PAC 3, CommonLook PDF Accessibility Software, European Internet Inclusion Initiative's PDF checker, and WebAIM's WAVE. These tools do not assist the user to remediate the accessibility issues. The author/user has to rely on other remediating tools or manually add accessibility markup in the source file. Adobe Acrobat Pro and PDF Accessibility Validation Engine (PAVE) are the two tools that can be used to both check and remediate accessibility issues.

4 Issues with Current Remediation Solutions

Existing tools for PDF accessibility have limitations and challenges that limit a smooth user experience with the tool. In this section, the major issues related to Adobe Acrobat Pro and the PAVE tool (the two tools that do remediation, not only evaluation) are discussed, and our potential solutions for tools of the future are described. We start by going deep in our description of identifying solutions to two of the most common problems - reading order and table tagging.

4.1 Reading Order

4.1.1 Problem

Screen readers rely on the reading order set in the document to read out the content. If the reading order is not set, the screen reader just uses the underlying order of the content, which depends on how the PDF was generated. This can be particularly difficult for users if the PDF has more than one column layout. The screen reader may read the first line of the first and second column together, which frustrates the user. Therefore, setting a reading order is very important for a screen reader to work effectively. Currently, both Adobe Acrobat Pro and the PAVE tool have a similar way of setting the reading order: the user has to tag each element of the paper in the proper reading order.

4.1.2 Potential Solution

Tagging the reading order of a document needs to be more efficient and intuitive. One potential solution is to mimic the natural gesture of the user tracing the reading order in a document. In case of a two-column layout format, the user might draw a straight line from the start of the first column paragraph through to the end of the first column using the mouse cursor. The same gesture could be repeated for the second column and subsequent pages. We anticipate that this would significantly reduce the time it would take to set the reading order compared to existing methods.

The user can redraw or alter the line to change the reading order of the page, with Fig. 1 showing how the user could draw the line and Fig. 2 showing how the application could provide notification to the user of the new reading order to ensure that it is what they intended. Another way of setting the reading order is to read out the contents of the page to the tool to set the reading order of the paper. This may prove useful for those who have no knowledge using the various tags.

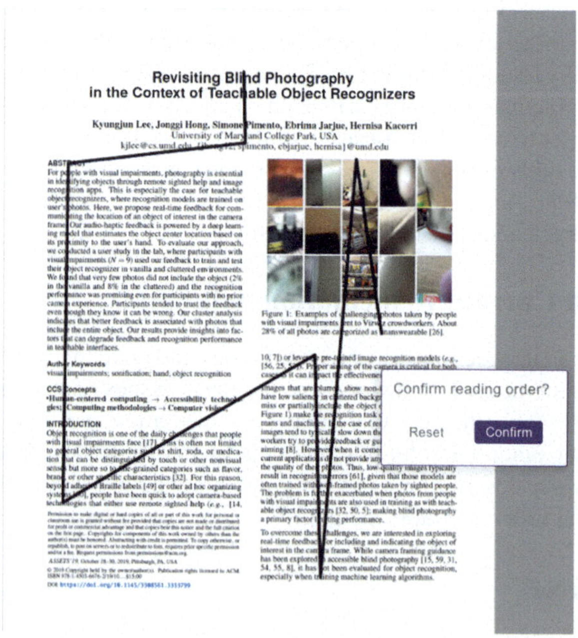

Fig. 1. An idea of how the user can set the reading order of the page by drawing vertical lines using a mouse

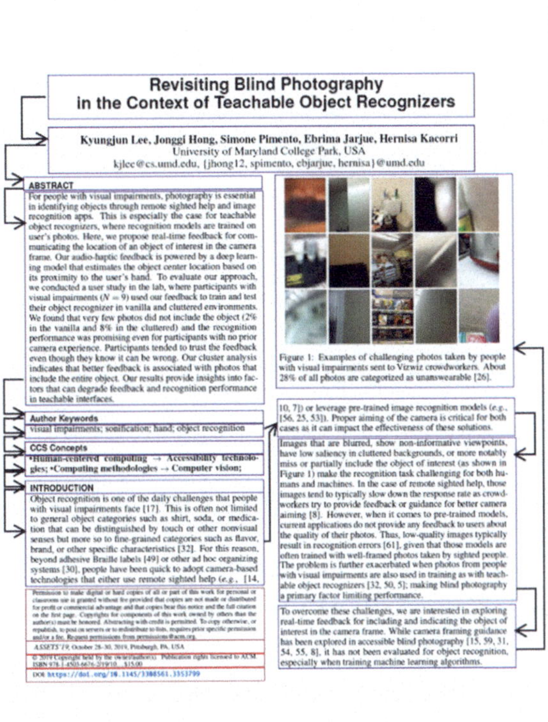

Fig. 2. The lines drawn by the user are now set as the reading order by the tool

4.2 Tagging Tables

4.2.1 Problem

Manually Tagging a table is particularly cumbersome and time consuming since it requires the user to tag each and every cell of the table and group the row and column headers. It also requires a basic understanding of the tags related to a table like <th>, <tr>, and <td>. Adobe Acrobat Pro lets the user group all the table data inside the table row tag. The table headers are also grouped inside the table row tag. All these are nested inside the table tag. For example, a simple four-column table with headers and a single row of data will look like Fig. 3 in Adobe Acrobat Pro.

Scaling these nested tags for complex tables will be time consuming and hard to track. The amount of time taken to tag the paper depends upon the number of tables present in the document and the size of each table.

4.2.2 Potential Solution

The PAVE tool (Fig. 4) has a more intuitive way of handling the table editor. The table editor has a visual representation of the table. The user has to set the number of rows and columns of the table and highlight each cell of the table and the tool automatically tags

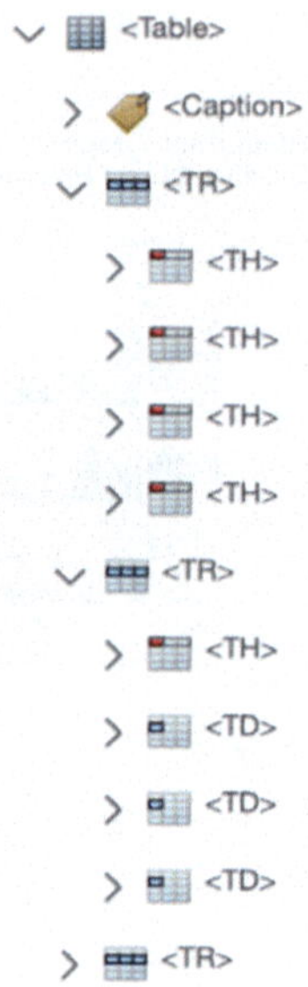

Fig. 3. A screenshot of Adobe's approach of tagging a table

them. This is a novel way of tagging the table as compared to Adobe's approach. The next step would be employing computer vision techniques enabling the tool to be intuitive enough to identify and tag the rows, columns and each cell of the table automatically. This may greatly reduce the time and effort to tag a table.

4.3 Auto Tag Feature and Retagging

An auto tag feature is available in both Adobe Acrobat Pro and PAVE, but they often tag everything in the document as "paragraphs" or <p> tags. In theory, the tools tag the entire document which causes them to pass the PDF accessibility checker, but some of the tags may not be appropriate depending on the context. The tools may misidentify tags thus requiring human supervision where the user has to re-tag some of the tags which were tagged by the tool. If this issue is not corrected, a screen reader will not be able to distinguish between the various heading levels, links and paragraphs.

Currently, PDF tagging and repairs are lost if a PDF needs to be corrected and re-exported from a source program/file. The PDF has to be tagged all over again even if a very small change has been made in the source file as the metadata is often not preserved due to the compatibility of content authoring tools and the operating system it runs on. One potential solution is to save the meta-data layer of all the tags and corrections as a template, with the help of machine learning the tool can allow the template to be reapplied to the document post-correction by matching the content and the structure. It would also identify the changes (grammatical corrections or inclusion of a few words) made to the document so that they could be repaired as well. This could reduce the need for the user to make versions of a PDF accessible over and over thus saving time and effort.

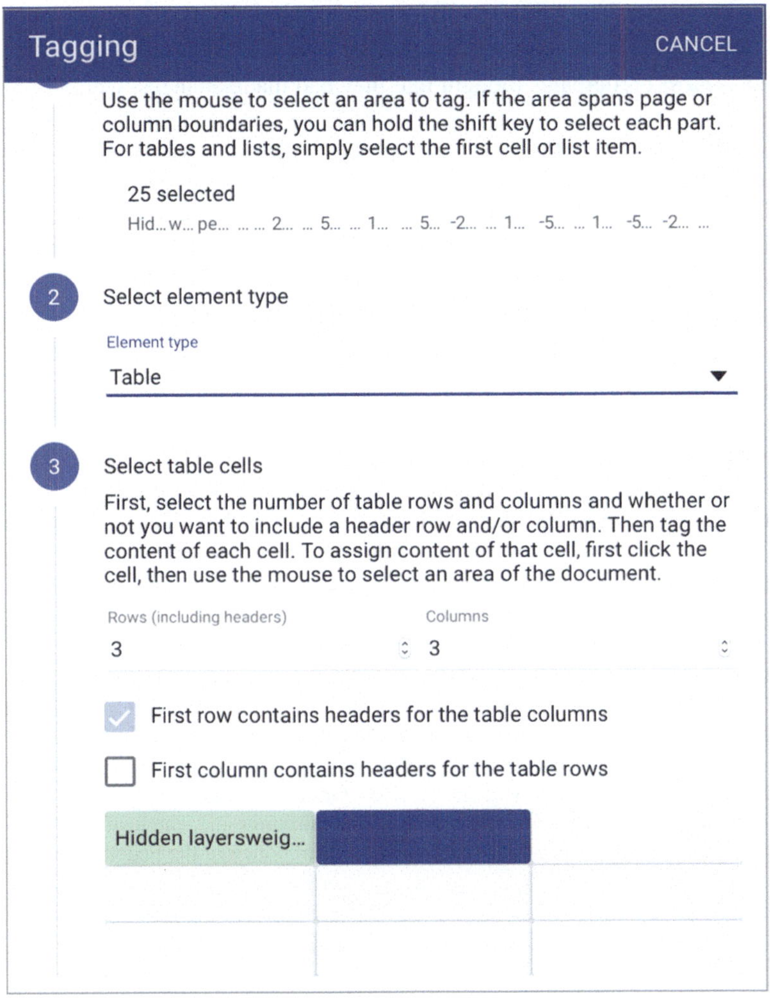

Fig. 4. A screenshot of PAVE's visual approach for tagging a table

4.4 User Experience

Participants from previous studies (Brady et al. 2015; Jembu Rajkumar et al. 2020) mentioned that both Adobe Acrobat and PAVE are not very user friendly. Depending on the version of the Acrobat Pro tool, some features in the software are not turned on or hidden by default like the accessibility tool kit which is found under the "More tools" button.

After including the accessibility tool kit in the current version of Adobe Acrobat Pro, the left pane consists of options like Articles, Tags, Order, Signature, Layers and 7 other options. By default, only 3 options are displayed on the pane. There are no signifiers or discoverability as to how to add more options on the pane. To see the list of tags in the document, the user has to go to the "Tags" option which is hidden in the left pane. In the study, the PAVE tool was also found to not be user friendly (Jembu Rajkumar et al. 2020). Users were not aware of the process of overriding a tag which was automatically tagged by the tool—most participants thought that they had made changes, which in fact were not saved.

The overall user experience could be improved with both tools by easing the learning curve and assisting the users who have limited to no knowledge of PDF accessibility. The tools should be able to simplify the process of tagging the document and intuitive enough to let the user be notified and fix the issues wherever tool is unable to fix. Complex workflows, and complicated visualisation of the tags should be simplified as much as possible to improve usability and smoothen the learning curve of the tool.

5 Conclusion

In this paper, we have discussed the existing literature on PDF accessibility and current tools for evaluation and remediation. We have also described our vision for remediation tools of the future, for content contributors who have no knowledge of PDF tags and accessibility. We need tools that automate the entire PDF tagging process and require minimum human supervision and expertise. This way, inaccessible PDFs are made accessible with minimal user effort.

Acknowledgements. The work reported in this publication was supported, in part, by grant number 90RE5027 (Universal Interface & Information Technology Access RERC) and 90REGE0008 (Inclusive ICT Rehabilitation Engineering Research Center), from the National Institute on Disability, Independent Living, and Rehabilitation Research, U.S. Administration for Community Living, Department of Health and Human Services. Grantees undertaking projects with government sponsorship are encouraged to express freely their findings and conclusions. Points of view or opinions do not, therefore, necessarily represent official policy of the Federal government.

References

Bigham J, Brady E, Gleason C, Guo A, Shamma D (2016) An uninteresting tour through why our research papers aren't accessible. In: Proceedings of the 2016 CHI conference extended abstracts on human factors in computing systems, San Jose, CA, US, 7–12 May 2016

Brady E, Zhong Y, Bigham J (2015) Creating accessible PDFs for conference proceedings. In: Proceedings of the 12th web for all conference, Florence, Italy, 18–20 May 2015

Itext (2019) Do you know how many PDF documents exist in the world? itextpdf.com/en/blog/technical-notes/do-you-know-how-many-pdf-documents-exist-world. Accessed 15 Oct 2019

Jembukumar A, Lazar J, Jordan JB, Hutter H, Darvishy A (2020) PDF accessibility of research papers: what tools are needed for assessment and remediation? In: Proceedings of the 53rd Annual Hawaii International Conference on System Sciences, pp 4185–4194

Lazar J, Allen A, Kleinman J, Malarkey C (2007) What frustrates screen reader users on the web: a study of 100 blind users. Int J Hum Comput Interact 22(3):247–269

Lazar J, Churchill E, Grossman T, Van der Veer G, Palanque P et al (2017) Making the field of computing more inclusive. Commun ACM 60(3):50–59

Nganji J (2015) The portable document format (PDF) accessibility practice of four journal publishers. Libr Inf Sci Res 37(3):254–262

Tomlinson SM (2016) Perceptions of accessibility and usability by blind or visually impaired persons: a pilot study. In: Proceedings of the 79th ASIS&T annual conference, Copenhagen, Denmark, 14–18 October 2016

WHO (2018) Vision impairment and blindness. World Health Organization. www.who.int/en/news-room/fact-sheets/detail/blindness-and-visual-impairment. Accessed 17 Dec 2019

Designer Attitudes to Accessible Information Provision on a Bus Route Map: Focus Group Discussions

G. Lee(✉), S. Westland, and T. Tang

University of Leeds, Leeds, UK
{ml13g31,S.Westland,T.X.Tang}@leeds.ac.uk

Abstract. Designers create information provision formats in the real world. They are commonly regarded as problem solvers. However, literature reveals that designers do not design information/products in an inclusive way and suggests various reasons for this. Designers continue to provide inaccessible information and seem not to consider various information users, especially vision and colour vision impaired people. Therefore, we implemented research to explore concrete factors and reasons why designers consistently continue to create inaccessible information even though previous researchers have already identified problematic factors. Focus group interviews were conducted with ten doctoral design students. It was revealed that these design participants have little knowledge of how to use design elements for target users, applied a subjective outlook for design selection, had a lack of design education and project experience, and used inappropriate information formats when searching for relevant information. Designers attitudes and values towards inclusive printed information practice were a particular focus of this study.

1 Introduction

Freedom of Information (FOI) is a fundamental and universal human right according to the United Nations Educational, Scientific and Culture Organisation (UNESCO 2017). However, Yet inaccessible information provision is spread around us.

Information is often inaccessible for disabled people, particularly for visually impaired people. Most visually impaired people face a number of additional difficulties compared to other groups of disabled people when accessing information (Playforth 2003; RNIB 2006). Interest in provision for those with disabilities has increased among professionals in design and communication, and so notions of access awareness have gained importance for these occupational groups (Gieben-Gamal and Matos 2017).

Various scholars (Roth 1999; Forlizzi and Lebbon 2002; Cornish et al. 2015), however, point out that print-based graphic/communication design particularly has problems in relation to accessibility. They also argue that it is an under-represented research area compared to other design practices. One reason for accessibility problems put forward by Cornish et al. (2015) is that in the print-based graphic area, users cannot modify the appearance of a proposed printed information source during the design process. This in effect means that the producers create or design information formats and material by

P. Langdon et al. (Eds.): CWUAAT 2020, *Designing for Inclusion*, pp. 182–191, 2020.
https://doi.org/10.1007/978-3-030-43865-4_19

relying on their own design knowledge, intuition or design skills in such tasks without accessing an essential element of user input. Designers frequently occupy such real-world information provision roles. In the contemporary design context, designers generally tend to be regarded as problem solvers (Sparke 1983; Lawson 2004). In an inclusive design context, they are engaged in promoting and delivering the design solution (Dong et al. 2015). However, existing research reveals that there are indeed challenges which prevent designers from designing information with user-centred design principles in mind. These challenges include designers' being intuitive (Wilkinson and Angeli 2014) and creative (Clarkson et al. 2003), a lack of user data (Forlizzi and Lebbon 2002), the belief that printed information is transitory (Roth 1999), the mistaken belief that designers would learn about users and approach their work with a user-driven mindset (Vredenburg et al. 2001), and the belief that inclusive design is less relevant to communication and interface design (Cassim and Dong 2005). Based on the above findings, the following research question and aim were adopted:

- Research question: why do designers consistently continue to create inaccessible information even though previous scholars have already identified this as a problem and identified problems that result from them doing so?
- Aim: to identify why there is a gap between what users need and what designers are providing.

It may be that without knowing about how designers think and assessing what they know, it will be challenging to provide appropriate suggestions for them to change their attitudes and values regarding more inclusive design. Therefore, we believe it is important to understand the gap between what design participants in our study predict about the needs of vision and colour vision impaired people, and what vision and colour vision impaired people actually do need as information users.

2 Methods

2.1 Participant Characteristics

A total of 10 PhD design students (four for an initial and six for a subsequent group session) were invited to volunteer to take part in focus groups. They were assigned a capital letter from A to J to identify them. They were aged from 24 to 32, and there were five males and five females. The number of participants comprised an adequate sample size for a focus group interview as set out by Krueger (2002) and Smithson (2008).

Homogeneity of samples was also considered for the participant recruitment (Morgan 1988). All participants were studying doctoral design degrees in information, colour, or fashion at the highest level of design education. In addition, two types of individual were mixed together in each group session: (1) those having experience of design practice, design education, or research experience and (2) those not experienced in the design area prior to commencing a PhD (Table 1).

Table 1. Participant information

Participant	PhD specialisation	Design experience prior to PhD (years)	Gender
Initial focus group interview			
A	Information	N/A	M
B	Information	Graphic design (1)	M
C	Information	Design teacher (1)	F
D	Information	N/A	F
Secondary focus group interview			
E	Colour	Design lecturer and graphic designer (7)	M
F	Colour	Graphic design freelancer (3)	M
G	Colour	N/A	F
H	Colour	N/A	F
I	Fashion	Design researcher (2)	F
J	Information	N/A	M

2.2 Research Procedure

In an initial phase (as part of an earlier design study) four prototypes of accessible bus route maps were created by one of the authors of this study, taking detailed account of vision and colour vision impaired people's first-hand experience and their opinions in an iterative design process. This involved conducting face-to-face interviews (both unstructured and semi-structured), email interviews, and focus group sessions conducted with eleven volunteers of target group users. Informants included a disability expert (former disability journalist) with vision impairment, four other participants with vision impairment, a participant with both colour and vision impairment, and five red-green colour-vision-impaired participants.

In the following stage, in order to investigate designers' assumptions, predictions and difficulties, two focus group sessions were implemented during April and June in 2019. The first focus group interview lasted about 50 min and the second about 40 min. All focus group sessions were digitally recorded and transcribed.

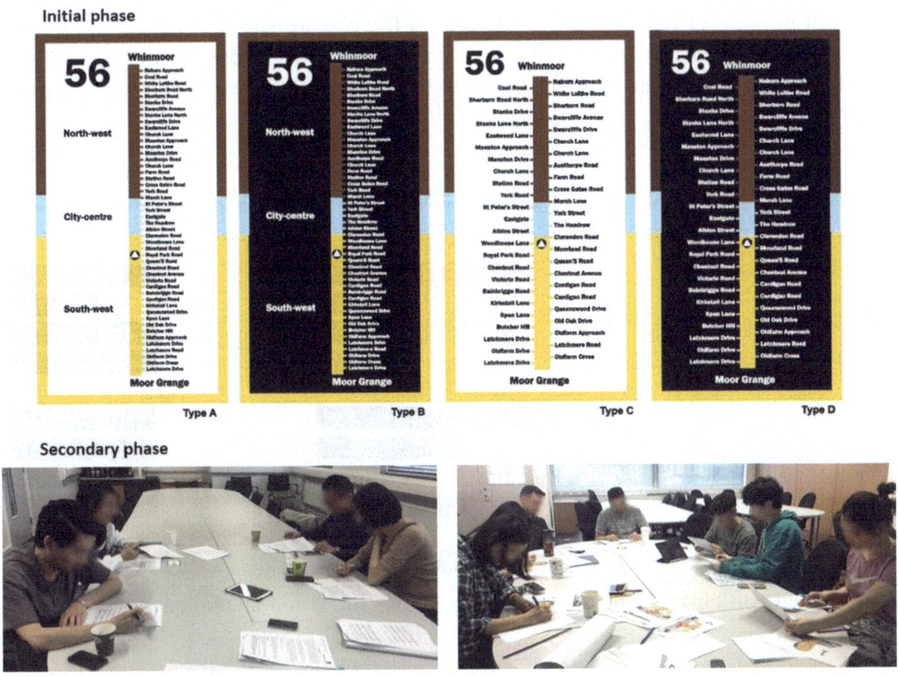

Fig. 1. Two steps in the experimental research process in this study

2.3 Data Analysis

Thematic analysis was adopted for analysing qualitative data. The collection of data was coded using an inductive approach. Thomas (2006) refers to the inductive approach as meaning that themes, concepts and models emerge from raw data interpreted by researchers. There were four themes covered during the group sessions: legibility and suggestions for colours, designers' subjective outlook, lack of education and research experience, and need for a designer friendly tool and information format. The themes are discussed in detail in the following section.

3 Findings and Discussion

3.1 Legibility and Suggestions for Colours

Colours improve visual images in terms of perception (Pettersson 2015). The use of effective colour schemes in information provision may be more important for people with visual impairments and colour vision deficiency than for those without such difficulties. Colour contrast may be a crucial issue here. In order to examine designers' knowledge of the use of colour for vision and colour vision impaired people, design participants were asked to suggest colour coding as a part of information legibility for both colour and vision impaired users. For this task, one of the researchers in this study converted the four prototype design samples (Fig. 1) into grey mode using the program Adobe Photoshop in advance. These were shown to the design participants during their group session.

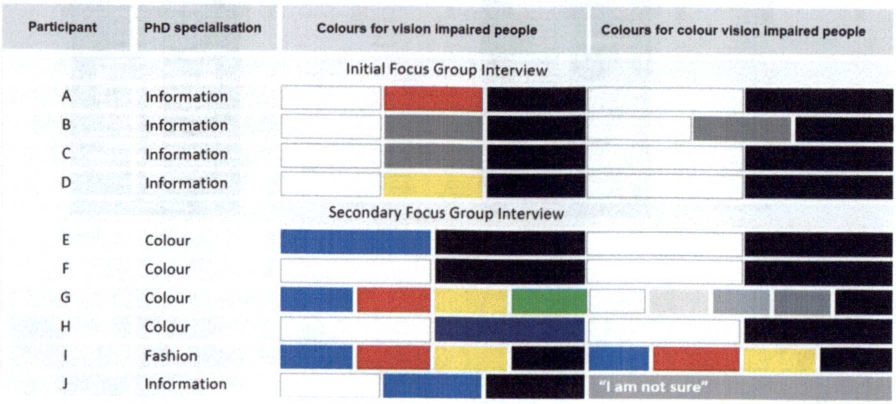

Fig. 2. Design participants' colour coding suggestions for vision and colour vision impaired people respectively

In terms of colour suggestions for people with vision impairment, participant H said "in my mind, I will just use black and white colours for the design because they do not mind what colours we use, they just want to read it clearly. We can just add some colourful logos for small details. We can choose the main colour, black and white". Participant E mentioned that "in terms of colours, I guess I use a high contrast for colours. I am not really sure about colour for vision impaired people".

When asked about colour suggestions for colour blind information users, participant J said that "they see certain colours looking quite similar. I am not real sure what colour combination to avoid for colour blindness, so I do not really know". Participant E added "I am not sure if colour blind people cannot see black".

It was found that all design participants have difficulty and also little knowledge in terms of using colour coding for various user groups who face difficulties in seeing and distinguishing colours. When discussing colour, the desinger considered only or mainly colour blindness despite being asked to consider both visual impairment and colour vision impairment. Figure 2 shows the colour suggestions by designers for visual legibility. Despite making colour-coding suggestions, they did not seem to think in-depth about the difficulties faced by vision impaired people in seeing/distinguishing colours.

3.2 Designers' Subjective Outlook

After the colour suggestion stage, the coloured printed prototypes of the bus route map were shown to design participants in their four forms (Fig. 1). Participants were asked to select which type of design would be most and least preferred by vision and colour vision impaired information users. The designs selected by design participants were different from those chosen by these information users. Only one design participant selected design type B – the design most preferred by the users. Design participants also found it hard to guess the least preferred design selected by the users (Table 2).

Table 2. Predictions of designers regarding vision/colour vision impaired users' most and least preferred prototypes (bold)

Participant code	What designers think is the most preferred	What designer think is the least preferred
A	A	**C**
B	C	A
C	A	D
D	**B**	**C**
E	A	D
F	A	D
G	C	B
H	A	D
I	A	C and D
J	A	D

During both group sessions, it was repeatedly observed that most of the design participants talked about their own preference rather than carefully considering what target groups of users would choose. For instance, participant E stated "I prefer [...] A. A and C are quite similar. Others are messy with too much information. A is more clearly-organised", then the others similar characteristics were revealed by other participants as well. For instance, participant J said "I think that's D. Yeh, just because I do not like it. Listed side to side". In addition, participant F added "I do not like B".

Their attitude was emphasised by frequent use of the first-person pronoun 'I' and the first-person possessive 'my', and utterances of the form 'I prefer to [X]', or 'I like [X]'. Similar characteristics were found by Lee et al. (2019) where design participants oftentended to be distracted from a set task during a design experiment. it was found that participants with a design background focused upon what they preferred and felt at the moment rather than seeing a task objectively. This characteristic of designers may impact on their designs reducing their orientation towards users.

3.3 Lack of Education and Research Experience

Authors have pointed out that there is little evidence of well-organised inclusive design courses in the design curriculum (Ho et al. 2011), and there are difficulties in teaching inclusive design for various reasons (Dong 2010). The design participants in this study, none of them had been taught design for a range of users at different cognitive and physical levels during the course of their education, even though they were now studying design at the highest level of design education. Apart from one participant (Participant D – whose PhD was based on inclusive information and environments for vision impaired people), they also had no experience of design or research projects taking such users into consideration. It is noteworthy that participant D was the only participant to correctly identify users most and least preferred design prototypes. This could serve as evidence that lack of experience in education, design research and projects in this area may be one factor that causes designers' to produce inaccessible designs.

An experiment using 10 design participants may be small for generalisations. However, what we draw from the findings here is that designers do not have enough knowledge, education, and design experience about diverse types of information users. A lack of knowledge about users and a subjective reaction in terms of doing design tasks may lead them to design based on their own intuition with inadequate consideration for users. There is in fact a huge gap between what designers assume and the actual needs of target users.

3.4 Need for a Designer Friendly Tool and Information Format

An understanding of the information needs of designers themselves is one of the research areas in the inclusive design domain (Dong et al. 2015). Visual images with short descriptions were offered since designers have a motivation towards communicating visually using mostly pictures and colour-based graphics, and minimising use of text (Lofthouse 2006). Information presentation is preferred by designers when it is quick, accessible and easy to use, visual and stimulating, flexible and open-minded, concise, concrete but also related to design issues clearly and precisely (Goodman et al. 2007). Both of the focus group sessions in this project produced similar findings, revealing that design participants prefer to find short and summarised information based mainly on bullet points rather than finding information in a range of chapters or sections of guides or books. One of the participants (participant C) stated that he spends little time reading in order to find information.

Participants were notified by email prior to the focus group interviews that they needed to bring their own information search tools. Personal laptops, tablets, and mobile phones were used to obtain user information during the sessions. Participants were asked to search for information if they thought they needed it to design for vision and colour vision impaired people. Then they were asked to describe (1) actual information they needed to know during the task (2) any barriers and difficulties faced in terms of finding information.

As for the actual information needs, examples of responses included "I would need to know the information regarding their actual problems. What kind of problems they have/what help they need/what design would be effective for them/the main problems when they faced some design" (Participant I). Other participants expressed a need to know "what colour combinations are appropriate to use for people with colour blindness and the desire for a list of design guidelines on how to design for visual impairment like text, size" (Participant J). Participant H felt it would be useful to know "how they distinguish different colours in their everyday life".

Generally, designers do not have vision impairments. Thus, it may be difficult for them to know about and empathise with different types of information readers. However, from the responses given by design participant above, it may be that instead of providing general guidelines for making information more accessible in textually rich formats, providing information in an alternative format may be useful for the designers themselves. This might convey actual problems and emotional responses to inaccessible information experienced by the target information users in a format that is preferred by designers (colours and pictures with less text).

It was found that information reliability is the main worry among design participants. Some of them do not have confidence themselves in terms of searching for appropriate information. One participant said "I am just wondering if it is correct information or not. I think I need professional information but I am not sure" (Participant I). Participant G also highlighted concerns about "information reliability".

In terms of preferred types of information format, it was noteworthy that more than half of the design participants preferred to find information from conventional sources (paper based) rather than online and gave various reasons for this. Although it is inevitable that designers will use computers in the current era, participants were concerned about an unstable internet environment, low batteries on gadgets (tablets, mobile phones and laptops) and any bad effects on their eye sight from looking at electronic products. Participant A indicated that if well designed sets of information cards existed, she would like to have access to them. These results suggest the need for further research to consider the benefits and drawbacks of both types of information formats (conventional and technology based) to determine how to provide information for designers in an effective and efficient way.

In order to encourage designers to consider various types of users and create information that is more accessible to users, designer-friendly information sources and formats may need to be developed by and for designers themselves. This could help to change designers' attitudes, behaviour, and the value they place on providing accessible information for disabled, visually impaired and colour vision impaired people. Of course, designers may ultimately need to consult detailed guidance to comply with legislation and understand requirements in detail. However, designer friendly guidelines/formats such as information cards may help to communicate with, inspire and inform designers in the first place and enhance their ongoing commitment to providing accessible information.

4 Conclusions

To conclude, the findings in this study suggest that there is in fact a huge gap between what designers assume and the actual needs of target users. Moreover, designers do not have enough knowledge, education or design research project experience related to diverse types of information users such as visually impaired and colour blind users, lack of knowledge, education and experience related to users, and subjective reactions in terms of doing design tasks may lead them to design information based on their own intuition with inadequate consideration for users. This could be one of the main reasons for designers neglect or making insufficient effort to find information themselves in order to consider users' access needs. These findings during the focus group interviews with design participants need to be considered to develop a designer-oriented information format and communication tool, and they suggest the need for further research. In this way we may change designers' attitudes, values and practice.

References

Cassim J, Dong H (2005) DBA design challenge: engaging design professionals with inclusive design. ACM SIGACCESS Access Comput 81:3–8

Clarkson PJ, Keates S, Lebbon C, Coleman R (eds) (2003) Inclusive design: design for the whole population. Springer, London

Cornish K, Goodman-Deane J, Ruggeri K, Clarkson PJ (2015) Visual accessibility in graphic design: a client–designer communication failure. Des Stud 40:176–195

Dong H (2010) Strategies for teaching inclusive design. J Eng Des 21:237–251

Dong H, Mcginley C, Nickpour F, Cifter A (2015) Designing for designers: insights into the knowledge users of inclusive design. Appl Ergon 46:284–297

Forlizzi J, Lebbon C (2002) From formalism to social significance in communication design. Design Issues 18:3–13

Gieben-Gamal E, Matos S (2017) Design and disability. Developing new opportunities for the design curriculum. Des J 20:2022–2032

Goodman J, Langdon P, Clarkson PJ (2007) Formats for user data in inclusive esign. In: Stephanidis C (eds) Universal access in human computer interaction. Coping with diversity. UAHCI 2007. Lecture notes in computer science, vol 4554. Springer, Heidelberg

Ho DK-L, Ma J, Lee Y (2011) Empathy @ design research: a phenomenological study on young people experiencing participatory design for social inclusion. CoDesign 7:95–106

Krueger RA (2002) Designing and conducting focus group interviews. www.eiu.edu/ihec/Krueger-FocusGroupInterviews.pdf. Accessed 11 Dec 2019

Lawson B (2004) What designers know. Architectural Press, Oxford

Lee G, Westland S, Cheung V (2019) Colour communication challenges: exploring disciplinary divides. J Int Colour Assoc 23:25–35

Lofthouse V (2006) Ecodesign tools for designers: defining the requirements. J Clean Prod 14:1386–1395

Morgan DL (1988) Focus groups as qualitative research. Sage, Newbury Park

Pettersson R (2015) Information design 5: cognition. Revised ed. Institute for Infology. www.iiid.net/PublicLibrary/Pettersson-Rune-ID5-Cognition.pdf. Accessed 14 Dec 2019

Playforth S (2003) Resource disability portfolio. Guide 6: Inclusive information. Resource, London, UK

RNIB (2006) See it right: making information accessible for people. RNIB, London

Roth S (1999) The state of design research. Des Issues 15:18–26

Smithson J (2008) Focus groups. In: Alasuutari P et al (eds) The SAGE handbook of applied social research methods. Sage, London

Sparke P (1983) Consultant design: the history and practice of the designer in industry. Pembridge Press, London

Thomas DR (2006) A general inductive approach for analyzing qualitative evaluation data. Am J Eval 27:237–246

UNESCO (2017) Communication and information. Freedom of information. www.unesco.org/new/en/communication-and-information/freedom-of-expression/freedom-of-information/. Accessed 27 Nov 2019

Vredenburg K, Isensee S, Righi C (2001) User-centred design: an integrated approach with CD-ROM. Prentice Hall, Upper Saddle River

Wilkinson CR, Angeli AD (2014) Applying user centred and participatory design approaches to commercial product development. Des Stud 35:614–631

Author Index

P. Langdon et al. (Eds.): CWUAAT 2020, *Designing for Inclusion*, pp. 193–194, 2020.
https://doi.org/10.1007/978-3-030-43865-4

The manufacturer's authorised representative in the EU is Springer Nature Customer Service Centre GmbH, Europaplatz 3, 69115 Heidelberg, Germany. If you have any concerns regarding our products, please contact ProductSafety@springernature.com

Printed and bound by CPI Group (UK) Ltd, Croydon, CR0 4YY
22/09/2026
02221057-0001